Nutrition in Child Health

Based on a conference organised by the Royal College of Physicians of London and the British Paediatric Association

Edited by

D P Davies MD FRCP

Professor and Head of the University Department of Child Health
University of Wales College of Medicine, Cardiff

1995

ROYAL COLLEGE OF PHYSICIANS
OF LONDON

Acknowledgement

The publication of this book is made possible by the continuing and generous support of the Children Nationwide Medical Research Fund to whom the Royal College of Physicians is most grateful.

Royal College of Physicians of London
11 St Andrews Place, London NW1 4LE

Registered Charity No. 210508

Copyright © 1995 Royal College of Physicians of London
ISBN 1 86016 018 2

Typeset by Oxprint, Aristotle Lane, Oxford
Printed in Great Britain by The Lavenham Press Ltd, Lavenham, Sudbury, Suffolk

Foreword

It is a sad fact that nutrition has been a Cinderella subject in the
education of doctors. Long ago when I was an examiner for the
Diploma in Child Health I sometimes used to take an orange and a
couple of sugar lumps from the examiner's lunch table in order to
provide a talking point on a nutritional subject in the afternoon
orals. My co-examiners smiled tolerantly and thought me eccentric;
the candidates were rightly appalled as their knowledge of even the
most elementary facts was, by and large, appalling. More recently I
examined in the Membership and hoped that matters might have
improved. They had, but not much. Any question with a nutritional
flavour still created great anxiety and it was a struggle to extract the
information.

Why does this situation exist? Nutrition is clearly the bedrock on
which is built growth and health. It permeates every aspect of the
care of children from conception and before, through to adolescence and beyond. Indeed nutrition in childhood may influence
the emergence of diseases much later in adult life. Nutrition
requires knowledge of physiology, biochemistry and metabolism;
of many diseases and their management; of psychology, sociology,
epidemiology and economics; even of geography and cooking.
There could hardly be a more exciting subject. Perhaps it is because
it crosses the boundaries of so many traditional medical disciplines
that it is so often left to 'someone else' to teach at 'some other time'.
Perhaps it is also because others are there in hospital and community to ensure that the children get the right food containing
the right nutrients at the right time. Here I do not refer to Robert
Lynd's waiters but to our skilled and highly trained colleagues, the
dieticians. And how we rely on them. I was saddened when I asked a
usually very competent senior house officer (who had gained his
Membership) about the nutrition of a patient to be told that
the dietician hadn't had time to work it out yet. Sad that our

iii

dieticians were so overworked; even sadder that a member of my own profession felt unable to tackle the task. The fact that dieticians are specialists does not absolve the medical profession from acquiring knowledge.

When Professor Davies suggested that the whole two days of a paediatric conference be devoted to the many faces of nutrition in paediatrics and child health I was delighted. I was even more delighted to learn that a publication would result. Those who attended the conference will have tasted the feast; they and those who could not come will want to enjoy the rich diversity of the written contributions. They describe the state of the art and look to the future. No longer should any paediatrician—young or not so young—be able to shrug off nutrition as a dull subject, or fail to give a sound opinion of children's food. The advice of the waiter is to lift the cover and begin.

May 1995   JUNE K LLOYD
Paediatric Vice-President,
Royal College of Physicians
and Past President, British
Paediatric Association

Editor's introduction

In choosing paediatric nutrition as the theme for the conference on which this book is based, I was confident that it would have appeal, above all, to paediatricians and others involved in the care of children – whether in hospital, the community or in primary care. It is clear that both in the developed and the developing worlds, child nutrition has become an increasingly important issue: indeed it is possible that certain diseases that become apparent only in adult life might have some of their origins during fetal development and in early childhood. Nutrition in child health has given rise to a rich tapestry of research which is revealing some surprising and important results and the proceedings of this conference will therefore also be of interest to many adult clinicians and medical scientists.

This book, like the conference, has four parts that reflect the multidisciplinary nature and rapid increase in knowledge in the field of paediatric nutrition.

Part 1 concerns the nutrition of the normal infant. It includes chapters on the physiology of breast feeding, how the nutrient quality of breast milk affects the composition of the infant's brain and the structure and function of the brain's biomembranes: other chapters deal with the problems surrounding weaning, particularly when to wean and the nutritional constituents of weanling foods and, in an international context, whether such foods should be supplemented. The final chapter in this section outlines the opportunities in primary care for nutritional intervention studies and for providing education on nutrition in the home.

The significance of nutrition in the fetal and neonatal periods is the topic of Part 2. It includes chapters on how poor fetal growth presages cardiovascular and metabolic disease in adult life, and on the importance of early 'catch-up' growth in the growth-retarded newborn whose damaged gastrointestinal mucosa hinders the absorption of nutrients from the gut. Other chapters deal with the nutrition of the preterm infant and whether the nutrient quality of pooled breast milk collected from nursing mothers is adequate for normal growth and protection against infection; and how early diet might have a lasting effect on later cognitive function and on bone mineral stores.

Part 3 deals with the importance of nutrition in the sick and problem child. Intraluminal nutrients are particularly important to help the recovery of an inflamed and damaged gastrointestinal mucosa. In children with cystic fibrosis, meticulous attention to diet improves not only their general health but also lung function. In acute and chronic renal disease doctors and dietitians must be alert to adapting the energy, protein, water and electrolyte content of the diet to the biochemical disturbances to speed recovery and sustain growth. There are chapters on how to cope with feeding children with cerebral palsy, with behavioural eating problems and those that are thought to be suffering from food intolerance. The final chapter in this part covers the indications for and problems of parenteral nutrition in the child's home.

With such a broad subject as nutrition which interfaces with so many disciplines, room must be found for topics which, though not conveniently fitting any particular theme, nonetheless contribute to the mosaic of nutrition problems and challenges. Part 4 of the book is in this category:- how nutrition can be appropriately taught in undergraduate and postgraduate training programmes; the enormous handicaps carried by children in less developed countries as the result of malnutrition; and, finally, a view of the current state of nutrition in children and adolescents in 'The Health of the Nation' and in particular how poor diet in this age group acts as a risk factor for suboptimal health in childhood and a sower of seeds for the common western diseases of affluence in adult life.

I would like to thank all the contributors for the high standard of presentation of their papers at the conference and also for so promptly delivering their written chapters to make possible this important publication. I am also appreciative of the valuable assistance from the Publications Department of the Royal College of Physicians, particularly Mrs Philada Dann and Miss Diana Beaven.

June 1995   D P DAVIES
                                                                     Cardiff

Contributors

David JP Barker MD FRCP FFCM *Professor of Clinical Epidemiology in the University of Southampton and Director, MRC Environmental Epidemiology Unit, Southampton General Hospital, Southampton SO9 4XY*

W Michael Bisset MD MRCP(UK) *Senior Lecturer in Child Health, Department of Child Health, University of Aberdeen, Foresterhill, Aberdeen AB9 2ZD*

Ian W Booth MD FRCP *Professor of Paediatric Gastroenterology & Nutrition in the University of Birmingham, Institute of Child Health, The Nuffield Building, Francis Road, Birmingham B16 8ET*

Forrester Cockburn MD FRCP(Ed & Glas) *Professor of Child Health in the University of Glasgow, Department of Child Health, Royal Hospital for Sick Children, Yorkhill, Glasgow G3 8SJ*

Michael Cosgrove BM BMedSci MRCP(UK) *Lecturer, University Department of Child Health, University of Wales College of Medicine, Heath Park, Cardiff CF4 4XN*

Jonathan M Couriel MB BChir MA FRCP *Consultant in Paediatrics and Paediatric Respiratory Medicine, Booth Hall Children's Hospital, Charlestown Road, Blackley, Manchester M9 2AA*

Timothy J David MD FRCP *Professor of Child Health in the University of Manchester and Honorary Consultant Paediatrician, University Department of Child Health, Booth Hall Children's Hospital, Charlestown Road, Blackley, Manchester M9 2AA*

David P Davies MD FRCP *Professor and Head of the University Department of Child Health, University of Wales College of Medicine, Heath Park, Cardiff CF4 4XN*

John A Dodge MD FRCP FRCP(Ed) FRCP(I) *The Queen's University of Belfast, Nuffield Department of Child Health, Institute of Clinical Science, Grosvenor Road, Belfast BT12 6BJ*

Jo Douglas MSc *Consultant Clinical Psychologist, Department of Psychological Medicine, The Hospitals for Sick Children, Great Ormond Street, London WC1N 3JH*

Alan A Jackson MA MD FRCP *Honorary Consultant in Clinical Nutrition in Southampton University Hospitals Trust and Professor of Human Nutrition and Director of the Institute of Human Nutrition, University of Southampton, School of Biological Sciences, Biomedical Sciences Building, Bassett Crescent East, Southampton SO16 7PX*

John James MB MRCGP *General Practitioner, Montpelier Health Centre, Bath Buildings, Montpelier, Bristol BS6 5PT*

Alan Lucas MD FRCP *Head of Infant and Child Nutrition Group, MRC Dunn Nutrition Unit, Downhams Lane, Milton Road, Cambridge CB4 1XJ*

Jane Morgan MSc PhD SRD *Senior Lecturer in Nutrition, School of Biological Sciences, University of Surrey, Guildford GU2 5XH*

Ruth Morley MB *Senior Clinical Scientist, MRC Dunn Nutrition Unit and Associate Specialist, Department of Paediatrics, Addenbrooke's Hospital, Hills Road, Cambridge CB2 2QQ*

John Puntis BM MRCP(UK) *Senior Lecturer in Paediatrics and Child Health in the University of Leeds and Consultant Paediatrician, Peter Congdon Neonatal Unit, Clarendon Wing, The General Infirmary at Leeds, Belmont Grove, Leeds LS2 9NS*

Andrew Tomkins MB BS FRCP *Director, Centre for International Child Health, Institute of Child Health (University of London), 30 Guilford Street, London WC1N 1EH*

Alan R Watson MB FRCP(Ed) MRCP(UK) *Consultant Paediatric Nephrologist and Director of the Paediatric Renal Unit, Nottingham City Hospital NHS Trust, Hucknall Road, Nottingham NG5 1PB*

Brian Wharton MD DSc FRCP FRCP(Ed & Glas) *Director-General, British Nutrition Foundation, High Holborn House, 52-54 High Holborn, London WC1V 6RQ*

Anthony F Williams DPhil FRCP *Senior Lecturer & Consultant in Neonatal Paediatrics, St George's Hospital Medical School, Cranmer Terrace, London SW17 0RE*

Michael W Woolridge DPhil *Director, UNICEF's "UK Baby Friendly Initiative" and Lactation Physiologist, Institute of Child Health, Royal Hospital for Sick Children, St Michael's Hill, Bristol BS2 8BJ*

Contents

PART ONE

Nutrition in the normal infant

1 | Breast feeding and the infant human brain

Forrester Cockburn
*Professor of Child Health in the University of Glasgow, Department of Child
Health, Royal Hospital for Sick Children, Glasgow*

Mammals probably first appeared on earth about 250 million years
ago and placental mammals in the last 100 million years. In the
Oligocene period of about 30 million years ago primitive homin-
oids (tailless primitive apes) made their appearance. During the
last 40,000 years, *Homosapiens sapiens*, characterised by a large and
complicated brain, has evolved the complex society we know today.
During the last 10,000 years man has learned to cultivate plants
and to farm animals and fish for food consumption. After the
agricultural revolution came the industrial revolution, and with it
during this past century the practice of using modified bovine
milks and synthetic plant-based 'milks' to feed newborn human
infants. Has this practice of artificially feeding the infant *Homosapiens sapiens* been an evolutionary step forward or backward?

The fetal and infant brain

Neuronal development starts early in fetal life; by 22 weeks gestation
most neurones have formed and have migrated from their area of
origin in the subependymal regions to the cortical surface where
they will form grey matter. During the second half of pregnancy
these cells develop complex arborisations, and after birth there is a
rapid increase in the numbers of synaptosomes on these neurones.
There is a peak of glial cell division during the first six months of
postnatal life.[1] At birth the newborn term human infant brain
weighs about 350 g. During the first year brain weight increases
threefold to reach about 1,100 g. The cerebral cortex, composed
largely of neurones and astrocytes, increases its weight during the
first year by some 750 g. Table 1 shows the infant brain growth and
composition during the first year of life: 47% of the increase in
brain weight during the first year takes place in the cortex, and the
bulk of the dry weight of cortex is lipid, predominantly phospholipid. Sixty percent of the total energy intake of the infant during

Table 1. Infant brain growth and composition (first year of life).

	Increase	
	%	Weight (g)
Brain weight		750
Cortex	47	350
Cortex (dry weight)	35	125
Lipid	60	75
Phospholipid	65	50
Docosahexaenoic acid	8	4

the first year is utilised by the brain, and much of this energy is used to construct neuronal membrane and to deposit myelin. The fat from both human milk and infant formulas is not simply a source of hydrocarbon for energy production but is comprised of a series of complex structures necessary for the creation of cell membranes.

Phospholipids and neuronal membranes

Mammalian membranes, whether at the cell surface or forming part of an intracellular organelle such as a mitochondrion or peroxisome, are predominantly phosphoglycerols and unesterified cholesterol. In neuronal membranes there are also sphingomyelins (phosphosphingolipids) and cerebrosides (glycosphingolipids). Singer and Nicolson have proposed a 'fluid mosaic model' of membrane structure in which phospholipid is present as a bimolecular sheet, with fatty acids held in the interior of the bilayer and polar phospholipid head groups on the internal and external faces of the membrane.[2] This lipid bilayer provides a flexible and adaptable structure into which are inserted proteins and glycoproteins such as enzymes, transmembrane transporter proteins and receptors. The major membrane phospholipids contain two fatty acids and a substituted (amino) alcohol attached to a hydrophilic glycerol phosphate backbone.

The nature of the alcohol head group and the attached fatty acids has major effects on the functioning of the membrane.[3] Cerebral cortical neuronal membrane phospholipids are composed of phosphatidylcholine (PC), phosphatidylethanolamine (PE), phosphatidylserine (PS) and phosphatidylinositol. PC is known to confer a structural stability to the neuronal membrane,[4] while the carboxyl groups of PS function as ion exchange sites.[5] PS and PE have a particularly important influence on the distribution of protein molecules, including the enzymes involved in neurotransmission in the membrane.[4,6] Incorporation of proteins into the PS and PE-rich areas of membrane is critically dependent on the chain length, degree of unsaturation and hence configuration of the two fatty acids attached to each PE moiety.[7] The long-chain polyunsaturated fatty acid docosahexaenoic acid (DHA) is a major component of the PS and PE which form the synaptosomal areas of neurones. The polyunsaturated DHA of these moieties preferentially cross-links with proteins, and the degree of unsaturation conveyed by these molecules can mediate the activities of membrane-bound enzymes.[8,9] PS and PE at the inner aspect of the phospholipid bilayer have high concentrations of DHA; this arrangement is a major factor in promoting the rapid and repeated complex biochemical activities that allow neurotransmission to take place at neuronal synaptosomes.[7,3,10] DHA is also the predominant membrane fatty acid in the retinal photoreceptors allowing the rapid conversion of light energy into electrical impulses.

Organic bases such as choline, ethanolamine, serine and inositol which are attached to the phosphoglycerides affect membrane thickness, elasticity, porosity and the ability to support and transmit other molecules.[3] The control mechanisms responsible for the siting and distribution of the different phospholipids are unknown. Protein synthesis will cease if essential amino acid supplies are absent, but incorporation of fatty acids into membrane phospholipids proceeds with the substitution of other available fatty acids, thus altering membrane properties. Where there is dietary deficiency of polyunsaturated fatty acids (PUFAs) of the n-3 series (which includes DHA), n-6 fatty acids replace them; n-6 fatty acids include arachidonic acid (AA) and docosapentaenoic acid (DPA). In extreme fatty acid deficiency states both the n-3 and n-6 series may be replaced by the n-9 family of PUFAs including Mead acid and dihomo-Mead acid.[11] The insertion of alternative fatty acids may render the membrane metabolically unstable and more permeable to water.[12] It has been found in animal studies that in n-3 fatty acid deficiency states there is selective substitution of DHA in the phospholipid membrane by DPA.[13–15]

Essential fatty acids

Two essential fatty acids, linoleic acid (C18:2n-6) and α-linolenic acid (C18: 3n-3), are the precursors of the n-6 and n-3 PUFA,

respectively, and must be present in the diet. At birth, infant subcutaneous fat contains very little of these essential fatty acids.[16]
The adult human is able to synthesise AA (C20: 4n-6) from linoleic
acid and DHA from α-linolenic acid, but the pre-term infant and
probably the term infant in the first four months of life have either
inactive or relatively inactive enzyme systems required for the
conversion of essential fatty acids into their long-chain PUFAs
(LCPUFAs). The term infant's subcutaneous fat has a small reserve
of LCPUFA, but this is insufficient to supply the 4 g of DHA
required during the first year of life (Table 1).

Human and formula fatty acid composition

Human milk provides a ready synthesised supply of DHA and AA
while many current infant formulas contain little or none of either,
and in some there is insufficient α-linolenic acid precursor to allow
for DHA synthesis (Table 2). There is variation in human milk DHA
and AA content (Table 3): the proportion of DHA in the breast milk
of vegan women is lower than in fish and meat eating women, but is
still substantially greater than in cow's milk formulas.

Cerebral cortex phospholipid fatty acid content and the infant diet

Breast-fed infants have significantly greater concentrations of DHA
in their cerebral cortex phospholipids than infants fed current
infant formulas.[20] There is substitution of DHA by LCPUFA of the
n-6 series derived from linoleic acid. In infants over four months the
predominant n-6 LCPUFA which substitutes for DHA is DPA (C22:
5n-6 (J. Farquharson; unpublished observations). The preferential
replacement of DHA in the phospholipid membrane by DPA can be
seen from Figures 1 and 2. This selective substitution of DHA by
DPA, although reported in animal studies, has not hitherto been
identified in man.[13–15] Synthesis of both DHA and DPA from the
parent essential fatty acids, α-linolenic and linoleic, respectively, is
dependent on a series of elongases and desaturases, some of which
may not function in early infancy. It appears that the DHA content
of PS in cortical neuronal membranes is 'protected' because there is
less substitution by DPA than that found in PE. Rat brain preferentially incorporates preformed long-chain fatty acids from the diet
and not those synthesised from the parent essential fatty acids.[21]
Formula fed infants have greater concentrations of n-6 PUFA in
their brains than breast fed infants and significantly less DHA.
These differences were found in the brains of cot death infants up

Table 2. Essential fatty acids and some derivatives in human milk and formulas. Mean weight percentage of total fatty acid present in the milks available in the UK in 1986–87 (values for 1993 in brackets).

Fatty acid	Breast milk	SMA Gold cap	Cow & Gate Premium	Farley's Ostermilk	Milupa Milumil
C18: 2n-6 (Linoleic acid)	7.2	16.0	14.5 (11.7)	12.5 (20.0)	10.0
C20: 4n-6 (Arachidonic acid)	0.7	ND	ND	ND	ND
C18: 4n-3 (α-Linolenic acid)	0.8	1.5	0.4 (2.2)	0.4 (0.25)	1.1
C22: 6n-3 (Docosahexaenoic) acid)	0.4	ND	ND	ND	ND

ND = not detected

Table 3. Average fatty acid composition of mature human milk from women on different diets.

Fatty acid	Mature human milk				
	UK (a)	Vancouver (b)	Inuit (b)	Vegans (c)	Vegetarians (c)
C18: 2n-6 (Linoleic acid)	7.2	12.7	11.5	23.8	19.5
C20: 4n-6 (Arachidonic acid)	0.7	0.7	0.6	0.32	0.38
C18: 3n-3 (α-Linolenic acid)	0.8	0.6	0.5	1.36	1.25
C22: 6n-3 (Docosa-hexaenoic acid)	0.4	0.4	1.4	0.14	0.30

(a) Data from Ref. 17 and author's own analysis.
(b) Data from Ref. 18.
(c) Data from Ref. 19.

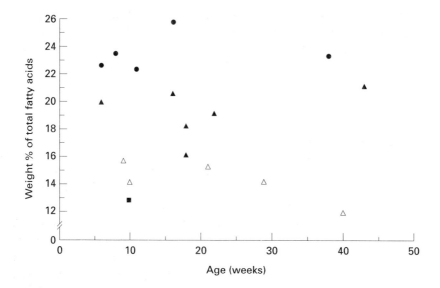

Fig. 1. *The docosahexaenoic acid content of infant cerebral cortex phosphatidyl-serine in infants fed breast milk or infant formula.*
(● = breast milk; ▲ = SMA; △ = CGOST (Cow & Gate Ostermilk);
■ = pre-term on SMA).

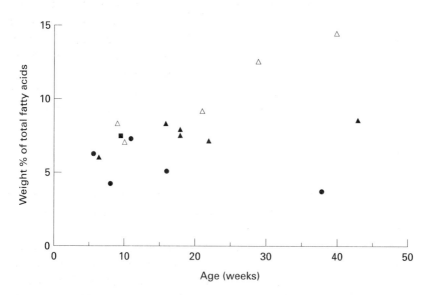

Fig. 2. *The docosapentaenoic acid content of infant cerebral cortex phosphatidyl-serine in infants fed breast milk or infant formula.*
(● = breast milk; ▲ = SMA; △ = CGOST (Cow & Gate Ostermilk);
■ = pre-term on SMA).

to 40 weeks after birth. In a pre-term infant studied by Farquharson (unpublished observations) there were significant quantities of Mead and dihomo-Mead acids in both the PS and PE fractions. These fatty acids are very unstable and must affect membrane function adversely.

Consequences of neuronal and retinal docosahexaenoic acid deficiency in infants

Pre-term infants fed human milk have higher developmental status at 18 months and a higher intelligence quotient in later childhood than those fed infant formulas.[22,23] They also have significantly different electroretinographic patterns indicating a delayed rod photoreceptor maturation in those fed standard infant formulas, and visual cortical functions are better in breast fed infants or in infants supplemented with DHA.[24] DHA supplemented and breast fed pre-term infants perform significantly better than standard formula fed infants on the Bayley mental scales.[25] It has been shown that term infants' visual responses at five months after birth correlate with erythrocyte DHA concentrations[26] and that human milk fed infants have better stereo acuity and matching ability at three years of age than do formula fed children.[27] In a recent review the British Paediatric Association Standing Committee on Nutrition has concluded that a factor present in breast milk, if fed for four or more months, is likely to be responsible for a greater cognitive function in breast fed infants,[28] and has suggested that DHA may be this factor. The balance of evidence now is that human milk conveys significant advantage to pre-term and term infants in terms of visual and cognitive functions compared to standard infant formulas.

Conclusion

The evolutionary processes which have allowed man to develop considerable intellectual achievements have taken many thousands of years. Paediatricians have observed during the last 100 years a move away from the natural human mammalian feeding processes in many countries throughout the world. Undoubtedly a need became evident during the last few decades of the 19th century that encouraged Pierre Budin in Paris and Justus von Liebig in Germany to develop artificial formulas which were free from pathogens and relatively digestible. This need arose from the enormously high mortality and morbidity found in infants fed raw cow's milk. From these early beginnings has developed a large infant milk formula industry.

A strong commercial drive to displace natural feeding of the human infant, together with altered family and work patterns, has resulted in very low levels of breast feeding in the UK and other 'developed' countries. The World Health Organisation has made strenuous efforts to redress the imbalance created by these pressures, but there is still a great deal that paediatricians and obstetricians can do to alert the population to the potential dangers of feeding synthetic formulas. There will always be a need for a few infants to have the benefits of artificial formulas when their own mother's milk or milk from a milk bank is unavailable. For this reason it is important that the best possible formulas be developed. In the meantime it would be prudent to encourage women to feed their infants themselves.

It is conceivable that the introduction of synthetic formulas during the past century for the feeding of the newborn human infant represents a major step forward in the evolutionary process; it is just as likely that it has predisposed the human infant brain to short-term defects in the efficiency of synaptic transmission and learning ability. There could also be longer-term effects which might predispose to adult neurodegenerative disease.[29–32] Both long- and short-term effects of this recent change in feeding practices warrant our urgent attention.

Acknowledgements

I gratefully acknowledge the work of my colleagues, Dr J Farquharson, Miss EC Jamieson, Dr K Abassi, Dr WJA Patrick, Dr AG Howatson and Dr RW Logan, quoted in this chapter, and of my secretary, Mrs Myra Fergusson, and of Miss Jean Hyslop, medical artist, for their help in the preparation of the text.

References

1. Dobbing J. The later development of the brain and its vulnerability. In: Davis JA, Dobbing J, eds. *Scientific foundations of paediatrics*, 2nd edn. London: William Heinemann, 1981: 744–59.
2. Singer SJ, Nicolson GL. The fluid mosaic model of the structure of cell membranes. *Science* 1972; **175**: 720–31.
3. Stubbs CD, Smith AD. The modification of mammalian membrane polyunsaturated fatty acid composition in relation to membrane fluidity and function. *Biochimica et Biophysica Acta* 1984; **779**: 89–137.
4. Cullis PR, De Kruijff B. Lipid polymorphism and the functional roles of lipids in biological membranes. *Biochimica et Biophysica Acta* 1979; **559**: 399–420
5. Cook AM, Low E, Ishijimi M. Effect of phosphatidylserine decarboxylase on neural excitation. *Nature-New Biology* 1972; **239**: 150–1
6. Fenske DB, Jarrell HC, Guo Y, Hui SW. Effect of unsaturated phosphatidylethanolamine on the chain order profile of bilayers at the

onset of the hexagonal phase transition: a ^{2}H NMR study. *Biochemistry* 1990; **29**: 11222–9

7. Salem N Jr, Kim HY, Yergey JA. Docosahexaenoic acid: membrane function and metabolism. In: Simopoulos AP, Kifer R, Martin RE, eds. *Health effects of polyunsaturated fatty acids in seafoods.* London: Academic Press Inc. 1986: 263–317

8. Orlacchio A, Maffei C, Binaglia L, Porcellati G. The effect of membrane phospholipid acyl-chain composition on the activity of brain β-N-acetyl-D-glucosaminidase. *Biochemical Journal* 1981; **195**: 383–8

9. Tanaka R. Comparison of lipid effects on K^+-Mg^{2+} activated p-nitrophenyl phosphatase and Na^+-K^+-Mg^{2+} activated adenosine triphosphatase of membrane. *Journal of Neurochemistry* 1969; **16**: 1301–7

10. Salem N. Specialization in membrane structure and metabolism with respect to polyunsaturated lipids. In: Karnovsky ML, Leaf A, Bolis LC, eds. *Biological membranes: aberrations in membrane structure and function.* New York: Alan R Liss, 1988: 319–33

11. Food and Agriculture Organisation and World Health Organisation. *The role of dietary fats and oils in human nutrition.* Report of an expert consultation. Rome: FAO, 1978

12. Stubbs CD, Smith AD. Essential fatty acids in membrane: physical properties and function. *Biochemical Society Transactions* 1990; **18**: 779–81

13. Bourre JM, Pascal G, Durand G, Masson M, *et al.* Alterations in the fatty acid composition of rat brain cells (neurons, astrocytes and oligodendrocytes) and of subcellular fractions (myelin and synaptosomes) induced by a diet devoid of n-3 fatty acids. *Journal of Neurochemistry* 1984; **43**: 342–8

14. Galli C, Trzeciak HI, Paoletti R. Effects of dietary fatty acids on the fatty acid composition of brain ethanolamine phosphoglyceride: reciprocal replacement of n-6 and n-3 polyunsaturated fatty acids. *Biochimica et Biophysica Acta* 1971; **248**: 449–54

15. Mohrhauer H, Holman RT. Alterations of the fatty acid composition of brain lipids by varying levels of dietary essential fatty acids. *Journal of Neurochemistry* 1963; **10**: 523–30

16. Farquharson J, Cockburn F, Patrick WA, Jamieson EC, Logan RW. Effect of diet on infant subcutaneous tissue triglyceride fatty acids. *Archives of Disease in Childhood* 1993; **69**: 589–93

17. Department of Health and Social Services. *The composition of mature human milk.* Report no. 12. London: HMSO, 1977: 21–2

18. Innis SM, Kuhnlein HV. Long-chain n-3 fatty acids in breast milk of Inuit women consuming traditional foods. *Early Human Development* 1988; **18**: 85–9

19. Sanders TAB, Reddy S. The influence of a vegetarian diet on the fatty acid composition of human milk and the essential fatty acid status of the infant. *Journal of Pediatrics* 1992; **120**: S71–7

20. Farquharson J, Cockburn F, Patrick WA, Jamieson EC, Logan RW. Infant cerebral cortex phospholipid fatty acid composition and diet. *Lancet* 1992; **340**: 810–3

21. Sinclair AJ. The incorporation of radioactive polyunsaturated fatty acids into the liver and brain of the developing rat. *Lipids* 1975; **10**: 175–84

22. Lucas A, Morley R, Cole TJ, Gore SM, *et al.* Early diet in preterm babies and developmental status at 18 months. *Lancet* 1990; **335**: 1477–81

23. Lucas A, Morley R, Cole TJ, Lister G, Leeson-Payne C. Breast milk and subsequent intelligence quotient in children born preterm. *Lancet* 1992; **339**: 261–4

24. Uauy R, Birch E, Birch D, Peirano P. Visual and brain function measurements in studies of n-3 fatty acid requirements of infants. *Journal of Pediatrics* 1992; **120**: S168–80

25. Carlson SE, Werkman SH, Peeples JM, Wilson WM. Long chain fatty acids and early visual and cognitive development of preterm infants. *European Journal of Clinical Nutrition* 1994: **48**: S27–30

26. Makrides M, Simmer A, Goggin M, Gibson RA. Erythrocyte docosa-hexaenoic acid correlates with the visual response of healthy, term infants. *Pediatric Research* 1993; **33**: 424–7

27. Birch E, Birch D, Hoffman D, Hale L, *et al.* Breast feeding and optimal visual development. *Journal of Pediatric Ophthalmology and Strabismus* 1993; **30**: 33–8

28. Standing Committee on Nutrition of the British Paediatric Association. Is breast feeding beneficial in the UK? *Archives of Disease in Childhood* 1994: **71**: 376–80

29. Horrobin DF, Manku MS, Hillman H, Glen AI, Glen M. Fatty acid levels in the brains of schizophrenics and normal controls. *Biological Psychiatry* 1991; **30**: 795–805

30. Soderberg M, Edlund C, Kristensson K, Dallner G. Fatty acid composition of brain phospholipids in aging and in Alzheimer's disease. *Lipids* 1991; **26**: 421–5

31. Brooksbank BWL, Martinez M. Lipid abnormalities in the brain in adult Down's syndrome and Alzheimer's disease. *Molecular and Chemical Neuropathology* 1989; **11**: 157–85

32. Pisacane A, Impagliazzo N, Russo M, Valiani R, *et al.* Breast feeding and multiple sclerosis. *British Medical Journal* 1994; **308**: 1411–2

2 | Breast feeding: physiology into practice

Michael W Woolridge
Lactation Physiologist, Institute of Child Health, Bristol;
Director, UNICEF's UK Baby Friendly Initiative

In the past, paediatricians have often felt powerless on how to advise women to overcome problems of breast feeding. The only practical advice to a mother presenting with her poorly growing infant was usually to feed more frequently (or, less sympathetically, to switch to artificial feeding). Increased awareness of the health benefits of breast feeding[1] now demands more substantive practical solutions to breast feeding problems, most of which are accessible if we equip ourselves with a sound up-to-date knowledge of the underlying physiology of lactation.

The commonest reason reported by mothers for discontinuing breast feeding remains a belief that they have insufficient milk for their infant.[2] Over the first four months of life apparent milk insufficiency is reported as frequently as the next five commonest problems combined. I would therefore like to focus in this chapter on an analysis of referrals to our breast feeding clinical support service (BCSS) in Bristol where, for the past three years, we have been conducting a Medical Research Council (MRC) funded project into identifiable breast milk insufficiency, with the aim of investigating its physiological basis.

Physiological basis for breast feeding problems

One overriding message is that there is an identifiable physiological basis to most breast feeding problems (including those of breast milk insufficiency), not a pathological one, and that such problems are rarely addressed by focusing on the mother in isolation. Invariably, the problem resides in the *interaction between the mother and her infant,* usually because of a failure to optimise some aspect of the feeding process, either physical or temporal.

Sixty-six per cent of all professional referrals to the clinic related to concerns over the mother's milk supply (Figure 1). Taking this group as a whole, such problems were readily correctable by routine methods in 85% of cases. Before considering the origins of these problems, however, some general issues need to be addressed.

First, a cautionary note to avoid one of the commonest pitfalls of assuming that where lactation is concerned 'humans are just another mammal'. As with all other mammals, human reproduction benefits from the reliability of placental nutrition of the fetus, followed by the type feature of all mammals, suckling the exterogestate fetus by the mammary gland. But there the similarity can stop. It is of some concern therefore that much of the common beliefs and myths about breast feeding come from the fields of veterinary and dairy science. The human mother, it must be emphasised, manages the process of lactation in an entirely different way from her non-primate mammalian counterparts.

Figure 2 shows the growth of an 'individual', born at 2.5 kg, whose weight increased in five weeks, whilst exclusively breast fed, to 10.5 kg. This 'superinfant' is, in fact, a litter of Springer Spaniel puppies, and is purposely misleading in order to make two

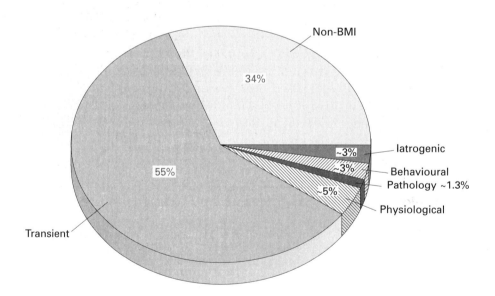

Fig. 1. *Analysis of referrals over $2\frac{1}{2}$ years to the breast feeding clinical support service (BCSS) at St Michael's Hospital, Bristol;* 66% of referrals are for apparent breast milk insufficiency (BMI) (34% non-BMI) and fall into five classes, of which the commonest is correctable transient insufficiency (55%).

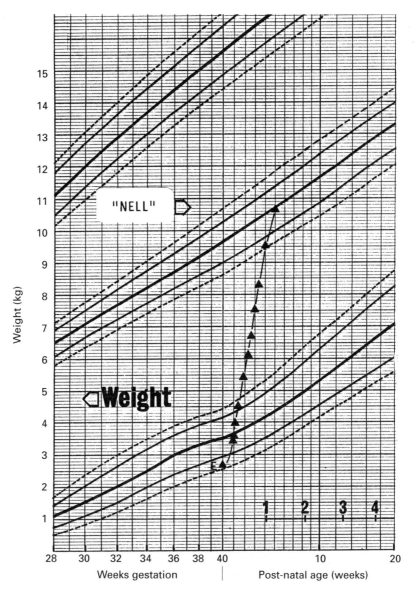

Fig. 2. *Combined weight increment for a litter of Springer Spaniel puppies whilst exclusively fed on bitch's milk* (growth from 2.5 to 10.5 kg in five weeks).

important points: first, the litter quadrupled their birth weight in just five weeks, a 'superhuman' feat—an animal about one-eighth the size of a human can achieve an eight times faster rate of weight gain whilst lactating exclusively, representing an apparent 64-fold difference in lactation efficiency. This aptly demonstrates that growth and development of the human newborn are typified more by their slowness than by rapidity (a point made many times before, most recently by Prentice *et al*[3]). But it demonstrates that in clinical trials of artificial alternatives caution should be exercised about accepting weight accretion as the sole outcome—other markers of neurodevelopmental progress and mid- to long-term health sequelae must also be considered, many of which (eg coronary heart disease) will be inaccessible to short-term clinical trials.

This illustration also highlights the fact that humans fuel the process of lactation differently. A domestic dog converts all her day-to-day nutrition into milk production. During the period when she is lactating, her own nutritional status is sacrificed in order to maximise the weight gain of her litter; if lactation was not programmed to be completed in a finite time she could ultimately jeopardise her own health. Fortunately, and contrary to the claims of Dugdale,[4] breast feeding is *not* a lethal condition for humans! To fuel the process of milk production, the bodies of lactating women juggle between daily nutrition and bodily reserves laid down during pregnancy, with the result that the infant is buffered from short-term fluctuations in dietary intake to ensure a relatively invariable diet (in macronutrient terms).[3]

A classical misconception that arose by generalising from mammalian to human lactation was that milk output by a mother was directly related to her nutritional status, from which the assumption was made that women on a low nutritional plane would be incapable of achieving a normal or adequate milk output. A summary by Prentice *et al*[5] of studies prior to 1975 derived from small selective samples of the population suggested that in the industrialised West well-nourished women typically exhibited milk outputs at or above 850 g/24 hours, whilst their less well-nourished counterparts in the developing world showed considerably reduced milk outputs, perhaps 650 g/24 hours. These data were seen to confirm a direct relationship between nutritional status and milk output.

As Prentice has pointed out, however, it became apparent from studies *after* this date, which employed larger samples with no obvious selection bias, that a yield of 750 g/24 hours was common to many different populations, demonstrating milk output to be largely independent both of the mother's ethnic origin and of her nutritional status (Figure 3). The present rationale for advising women to follow a balanced diet during lactation is therefore *not* to preserve either the quantity or quality of their milk output, but to protect their own health against micronutrient depletion.

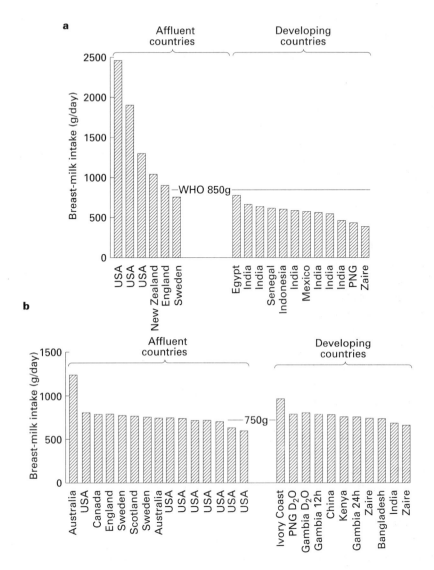

Fig. 3. *Breast milk intake data at three months of age.* **a.** data from studies prior to 1975, indicating limited sample sizes and selection bias; **b.** studies after 1975, based on larger sample sizes randomly selected, indicating a universal milk volume of 750 g/24 hours, irrespective of the mothers' origin (taken from Prentice *et al*[5]).

This discussion is relevant for two main reasons: first, because later I will make the assertion that infant appetite control is triggered by fat (or calorie) intake. Ineffective triggering of the infant's satiety mechanism will result in the infant crying and being unsettled after feeds. This might prompt an initial conclusion that a mother's milk quality is deficient, but it would be a fallacy to suggest that attempting to boost her dietary intake of fat would improve the quality. Variation in the fat content of milk is almost entirely a function of the efficiency of milk removal/delivery from the breast, with the fat content being improved by maximising milk transfer.[6]

Secondly, the solutions to most breast feeding problems are readily available, but it is necessary first to:

• re-evaluate our knowledge of 'classical' physiology—certain implications which should be self-evident have largely been overlooked; and

• attach greater significance to the regulation of supply by peripheral factors, which means embracing new areas of physiological knowledge.

Both of these can help dramatically in understanding and managing breast feeding problems.

Re-evaluation of 'classical' physiology

At least six separate stages in lactation can be identified (Table 1), although Stages 2, 3 and 4 are most relevant to clinical problems of milk production.

Onset involves 'disinhibition'

The factor which triggers lactation appears to be delivery of the placenta with the associated loss of the placental steroids, oestrogen and progesterone, from the maternal bloodstream.[7] The high levels of prolactin achieved during pregnancy are then allowed to exert an influence upon the mammary glands, and milk production begins through disinhibition.

However, the data given in Figure 4 demonstrate that milk production at five days post-partum is highly variable

Table 1. Stages of lactation

1.	Priming
2.	Initiation
3.	Calibration
4.	Maintenance
5.	Decline
6.	Involution

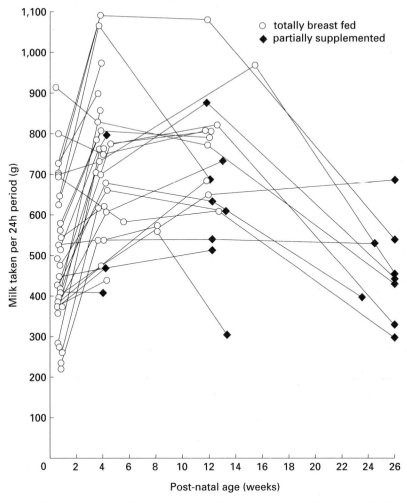

Fig. 4. *Normal data for 24-hour breast milk intake compiled from 30 individuals in Bristol.* The data reveal a range of 700 g between the highest and lowest intakes at all ages (five days, four weeks and three months). Breast milk intakes decline from three months when babies are supplemented with solids.

(200–900 g/24 hours). It is as if milk production gets underway without any reference to the baby's size. (In practice, placental lactogen is likely to exert some influence on milk production, which might be verified by comparing initial levels of milk output between monozygotic and dizygotic twins.) Over the next 3–5 weeks milk output is progressively calibrated to the baby's needs, in most cases building up to meet them ('up-regulation') but, in a few, 'down-regulating' to match the baby's needs.

In a proportion of women who present clinically it seems that this process of down-regulation may be irreversible during the current lactation. If, therefore, during the critical early phase of lactation the baby is offered calories from an alternative source (supplementary formula, for example), the breasts may calibrate their output at an inappropriately low level. In this way, peak milk output may never be realised.

This is a crucial aspect of physiology with important clinical implications: for example, it implies that if women encounter severe milk engorgement in the early post-partum period milk should be removed to minimise the potential to down-regulate supply to a critical level. It also means that a mother with a pre-term or small-for-dates baby, who must express her milk initially, should express up to her peak yield rather than to her baby's transiently limited needs.

Milk output is a two-stage process

The profile shown in Figure 5 was compiled from 16 studies of the milk intake of exclusively breast fed infants.[8] It indicates that milk output over time is a two-stage process: following initiation, milk output rises to about 700 g/24 hours by 4–6 weeks of age (rate of

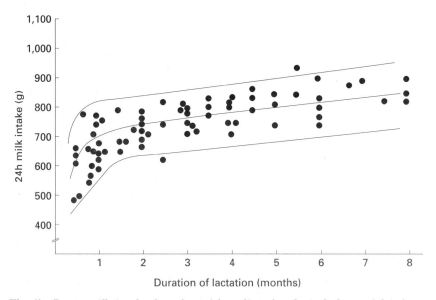

Fig. 5. *Breast milk intake data from 16 studies of exclusively breast fed infants.* Intake rises steeply to approximately 700 g/24 hours at 4–6 weeks, after which the rate of increase declines sharply to 4 g/week (compiled by Neville *et al*[8]).

increase, 175 g/week), after which it slows dramatically (rate of increase, 4 g/week) giving an impression of stabilising.

Clearly, milk intake does *not* directly match infant growth over this period. I believe that these data indicate that milk production reaches an asymptote. The apparent increase after six weeks is the result of several isolated points, one each from different studies. (It becomes increasingly difficult to find exclusively breast fed infants at 7, 8 and 9 months post-partum, and data collected from such infants may be less representative of the population as a whole.) So, following the initiation of milk production and calibration of milk output to the baby's needs, breast milk output stabilises and is maintained until some other factor causes it either to decline (fewer breast feeds offered) or to be depressed (caloric competition from weaning foods).[9]

The existence of this two-stage process raises the probability that different control factors are responsible for the initiation and calibration phase up to five weeks and during the maintenance phase from that time onwards. I contend that *on average* the milk intake of a singleton equilibrates at 750 g/24 hours from five weeks onwards, and falls from this level only under the influence of caloric competition from weaning foods.

This picture emerges from studies in Thailand, where the introduction of weaning foods typically starts early, usually by one month of age, which would signify that Stage 3 (calibration) runs directly into Stage 5 (decline) without an intervening period of stabilisation (Stage 4) free from the influence of weaning foods.[9] In contrast, data from the USA, where the introduction of weaning foods is often delayed because of cultural beliefs among dedicated breast feeders, show a different pattern, with weaning foods appearing truly to supplement gross intake.[10]

That 750 g/24 hours meets the needs of the average singleton from about five weeks onwards would seem to constitute a biological 'rule'. Although the infant is growing throughout this time, its energy requirements per kg body weight are falling, with the result that a constant milk supply is able to meet its needs for a major part of infancy. Milk output is not absolutely constrained as most women would be capable of producing 1,500 g/24 hours if they were able to suckle twins.

Karlberg[11] has modelled infant growth and identified three distinct growth phases. He suggests that a 'childhood' growth component cuts in at about 8–9 months of age. Its influence gradually overtakes the 'infancy' growth component. It may be that energy requirements increase again only as this happens. A cross-sectional compilation of data relating to the baby's changing energy needs (intake/kg) over the first year has suggested that they can be modelled by a U-shaped curve.[12] I suspect, however, that this curve may arise from a more linear decline over the first part of infancy to intercept a second rising line at 8–9 months, as suggested by Karlberg's growth model.[11]

A shift in control?

The picture which emerges, as yet to be confirmed, is that prolactin may play its predominant role in the early days setting the broad limits on milk output. Once peak milk output is achieved at around five weeks, control is then largely achieved by peripheral regulation. In recognition of this, two factors should be embraced and be given equal consideration with central maternal factors in the regulation of milk supply:

- autocrine control; and
- appetite control.

Both these factors are the ultimate regulators of supply during established lactation, and appetite control by the infant should be set alongside hormonal processes as being of equal importance.

Peripheral regulation of breast milk supply

There are several features of lactation which the 'classical' physiology does not explain. For example, it is not uncommon to meet women who are feeding exclusively on only one breast, having suspended feeding from the other breast. How can this happen? If the central hormones, which act on both breasts, were alone responsible, how can one breast switch off and ignore the central message whilst the other carries on as normal? This could happen only if a local peripheral factor was operating which is capable of overriding the central message. Such a factor has now been identified.

Autocrine control. Research, principally with goats, at the Hannah Research Institute, Ayr, Scotland, has identified a milk fraction synthesised by the mammary secretory cells which acts locally to inhibit the secretory output of those cells. During the interval between feeds its concentration builds up in the luminal space and is capable of inhibiting milk synthesis.[13] An equivalent factor has since been identified in human breast milk.[14] Slowing of milk synthesis as the breast refills, consistent with the action of an inhibitory factor, has been demonstrated using a novel imaging technique for making quantitative measurements of breast size.[15]

The clinical message is that if milk production is to be sustained, synthesised breast milk must be consistently and effectively removed. Unremoved milk is likely to exert a sustained inhibitory effect on milk production, and is likely to be the mechanism by which breast involution, the reversal of lactation initiation, is achieved.

Appetite control.   It has long been recognised that milk production is regulated by the process of supply and demand, with many people regarding infant demand as the key regulating factor.[16,17] This means that infants must be recognised as being capable of expressing appetite control, and I feel this should be considered along with hormonal factors in the regulation of milk supply.

Appetite control by the infant has been demonstrated in studies of bottle fed babies who have been shown to modify their volume intake in response to the caloric density of the formula given.[18] This process took up to 42 days to be fully expressed in artificially fed infants, but a more recent experimental study of breast fed babies suggested that they may be capable of regulating their fat intake on a much shorter time scale.[19] Twenty mothers experiencing problem-free breast feeding were asked to follow each of two alternative patterns of breast usage for one week prior to measurement of the baby's volume intake. The fat concentrations of pre-feed and post-feed expressed breast milk samples were measured to estimate the baby's net fat intake. The two patterns were either to offer both breasts at every feed or to try to feed exclusively from only one breast at each feed, switching breasts at consecutive feeds (order of presentation randomly determined). Neither pattern is recommended as a *fixed* strategy, as mothers are encouraged to be flexible, but they were implemented here for experimental purposes.

The experimental differences are best summarised by an analysis of variance comparing between-mother variance with that induced by the experimental treatment (Table 2). There were significant differences in 24-hour volume intake both between mother/infant pairs and as a function of the experimental treatment. In contrast, differences in the mean fat concentration of expressed milk samples were not consistent between mother/infant pairs although the experimental treatment produced consistent and significant differences. The pre-feed milk fat concentrations were routinely

Table 2. Two-way analysis of variance

Variable	Between mothers	Between treatments
24-hour volume	23.4 ($p < 0.001$)	21.9 ($p < 0.001$)
Mean fat concentration	2.9 (NS)	9.5 ($p < 0.05$)
Net fat intake	5.4 ($p < 0.05$)	0.1 (NS)
Index of emptying (%)	0.5 (NS)	20.1 ($p < 0.001$)

NS = not significant.

lower on the one breast per feed pattern, but substantially and significantly higher at the end of the feed. In marked contrast, the derived measure (net fat intake) showed significant variation between infants, but no difference as a function of the experimental treatment. The total absence of variation in the babies' net fat intake, despite significant variation both in the volume of milk taken and in the fat concentration of that milk, seems to provide strong evidence that the babies were actively regulating their fat intake. A measure of the consistency of milk, removal was calculated (the index of emptying (%)). This showed no predictable variation between mother/infant pairs, but it was the factor most specifically affected by the experimental treatment.

When these two areas of peripheral regulation are considered together, it might be concluded that the efficiency of milk removal (breast emptying) both *regulates supply* by effective removal of the autocrine inhibitory factor and *maximises milk quality*, in particular the fat concentration of the milk which is essential for effective triggering of satiety in the infant. Efficiency of milk removal is predominantly a function of the quality of mouth to breast apposition (positioning and attachment) and the duration of access to the breast permitted to the infant.

Lessons for clinical practice

Sound clinical practice must embrace these physiological principles as they provide an essential framework for understanding the basis of common breast feeding problems and also offer ready clues to their management. The majority of problems should be readily overcome by applying these principles, as I will now demonstrate by

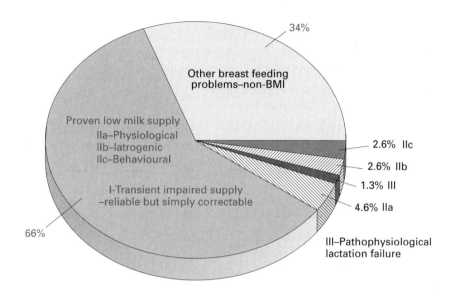

Fig. 6. *Case referrals to the BCSS for breast milk insufficiency broken down into five natural classes* (I: transient, unsubstantiated; IIa: physiological; IIb: iatrogenic; IIc: behavioural; III: pathological).

exploring the problems of genuine breast milk insufficiency undertaken in a clinical research study funded by the MRC.

Symptoms suggestive of breast milk insufficiency are the commonest cause for referral to the BCSS at the Bristol Maternity Hospital. Of the 1,088 referrals by health care professionals during a $2\frac{1}{2}$-year period, 705 received clinical consultations of whom 465 (66%) presented with symptoms suggestive of low milk output (Figure 6) (Table 3). No simple quantitative breakdown in terms of measured milk output has been found to suffice.

Apparent breast milk insufficiency

Referrals to the clinic presenting with symptoms of apparent milk inadequacy gave reliable clinical features in 96% of instances:

- slow or static infant weight gain or weight loss;

- unsettled infant behaviour contingent on feeding (crying after feeds, the baby feeding too long, or too frequently); or

- perceptions by the mother that her supply was not as good as it had been earlier (less sense of breasts being full, cessation of leakage).

Table 3. Classification of apparent milk insufficiency.

Class I—Unsubstantiated low milk supply
- Acquired, transient low supply: symptoms reliable but simply correctable by specialist physiological input and support.

Class IIa—Physiological low milk supply
Milk output 150–350 g/24 hours
- Intrinsic to mother, of NO identifiable origin.
- Unresponsive to therapeutic approaches including anti-dopamine agents (output >350 g/24 hours may respond to pharmaco-therapy).

Class IIb—Iatrogenic low milk supply
Milk output <450 g/24 hours
- Evidence of higher milk output at an earlier stage, but failure to sustain output due to mismanagement.
- Acquired, irreversible by six weeks?

Class IIc—Behaviourally induced low milk supply
Milk output <450 g/24 hours
- Induced by infant self-limiting intake at an inappropriately low level.
- Outcome of behavioural coping strategy in response to aversive stimuli, or aspects of feeding which infant unable to control (may be reversible by external intervention).

Class III—Pathophysiological lactation failure
Milk output typically <150 g/24 hours
- Intrinsic organic problem of maternal origin (eg agenesis of breasts during puberty, hypothyroidism).
- Dysfunction induced by peri-partum event (irreversible: pituitary necrosis (Sheehan's syndrome); reversible: retained placental products).

Class I: unsubstantiated low milk supply. The vast majority of such referrals (395, 85%) were resolved by offering individual specific help:

- advising on technical improvements to physical aspects of the breast feeding process;
- recommending ways to optimise feed management (frequency, duration, pattern of breast usage); and
- providing support and encouragement.

Most problems can therefore be regarded as being due to inadequate knowledge about breast feeding technique and on ways to improve matters. There is clearly scope for improvements in professional training in this key area, as the inability to correct routine problems of breast feeding will inevitably cause un-necessary supplementation of infants and overdiagnosis of 'breast milk insufficiency' as a clinical entity.

Class IIa: physiological low milk supply.   The rest of the referrals (70, 15%) for apparent breast milk insufficiency did not respond promptly to routine advice and support, so required further investigation. This was achieved by requesting the mother to undertake 24-hour test weighing at home on electronic scales.[20] Normal data have previously been collected on breast milk intake for infants in Bristol (Figure 4), from which centiles have been compiled for milk intake which are used as a local reference guide for evaluating *clinically* low milk output (Figure 7).

By far the larger group of women (approximately 13%) showed a milk output on or below the 10th centile (<450 g/24 hours) for the normal population. This percentage is accountable for in a population of clinical referrals, and such women may be regarded as exhibiting physiological low milk supply of no specific origin.

Several therapeutic strategies are available (adjunctive use of an electric breast pump, pharmacotherapy), but only if lactation was unresponsive to these approaches were women included in this class. For many women whose milk supply fell at the lower end of the normal range minimal supplementation was recommended, in order to sustain growth without diminishing existing milk supply, but the recognition of this should never constitute a reason to discontinue breast feeding—mixed feeding will continue to assure many of the growth benefits to the infant.

Our studies, however, have identified two further causes of low breast milk output within this class which would previously have been regarded as undersupply of maternal origin.

Class IIb: iatrogenic low milk supply.   The first, acquired irreversible low supply appears to result from excessive down-regulation of supply. Milk output at the onset of lactation, as described above, is calibrated to meet the infant's needs, a process which takes 4–6 weeks; after this it appears that a degree of flexibility in supply is lost. If supply is set at an inappropriately low level due to suboptimal management (this can include artificial supplemen-tation with formula), in a proportion of cases it does not seem possible to improve matters even by pharmacotherapy.

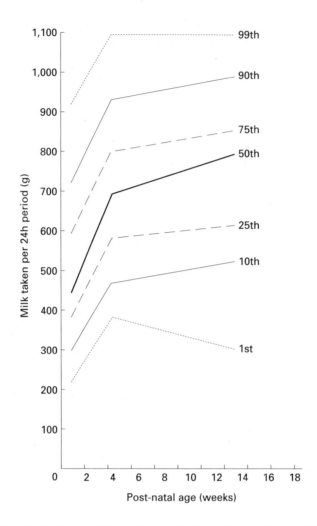

Fig. 7. *Centiles for breast milk intake compiled from 55 sets of normal data (Bristol and Oxford), used as a local reference guide for evaluating clinically low milk output* (assessed by 24-hour test weighing conducted by the mother at home on electronic scales[20]).

Class IIc: behaviourally induced low milk supply. The second new class may be termed acquired, behaviourally induced low supply caused by the baby adopting a behavioural coping strategy to avoid aversive events, for example, inappropriate use of force to latch a baby on to the breast, or excessive pressure to hold it there. Alternatively, the control which the baby would normally exercise over many aspects of ingestion may have been lost or overridden in some respect. Loss of breathing at any stage of ingestion invariably results in overt breast refusal, whereas loss of control over some aspect of feeding is more likely to result in a non-overt coping strategy such as a behavioural lack of persistence. The behavioural self-limitation of intake which can result may account for the condition described by Davies[21] as 'contented underfed babies'.

Several of these classes (IIa, IIb and IIc) may overlap and share aetiological factors. For example, milk oversupply (reverse of IIa), often associated with vigorous milk release and colic, might cause the infant to terminate feeds prematurely (IIc), opting instead to suck on a 'dummy'—in the long term this would cause a decline in supply which might prove difficult to reverse after a certain time has elapsed (IIb).

Class III: pathophysiological failure.   No more than 2% (9) of women presenting with apparent breast milk insufficiency had a genuine pathophysiology of milk production. Several rare causes, including mammary hypoplasia either at puberty or in pregnancy (absence of breast growth/enlargement), may manifest as absence of lactogenesis (absence of milk production post-partum). Two specific peri-partum events can have a catastrophic effect on milk synthesis:

- retained placental products, inhibiting lactogenesis; and
- necrosis of the anterior pituitary due to a hypotensive episode (Sheehan's syndrome).

The former is reversible when detected, but not the latter; both are likely to show in the immediate post-partum period.

Conclusion

Within a relatively large group of women who have genuine symptoms of low milk supply but no intrinsic problem, a small but significant proportion present with proven low milk output. There may be predisposing factors, but in many cases it is an acquired state arising through suboptimal management. Unless the causes are identified and promptly corrected, the acquired undersupply may become irreversible.

This discussion indicates that when a mother reports having insufficient milk to meet her baby's needs this should not be regarded as either intrinsic or irresolvable, but a state which may be reversed in the majority of cases. In the rarer cases where a clinical entity exists, the mother is likely to benefit most from being referred to a specialist breast feeding service where she should receive experienced advice and support. Unfortunately, very few referral clinics currently exist.

Our own clinical experience indicates that primary breast milk insufficiency is overdiagnosed to a marked extent (by both hospital and community health care staff). The fact that 85% of such crises are simply resolvable suggests that health care staff are not fully equipped with the essential skills necessary to manage breast feeding. This may be due to:

- the absence of any formal requirement to demonstrate an ability to manage breast feeding problems;
- the lack of emphasis on the apprenticeship method of skill acquisition (shadowing a mentor);
- the paucity of knowledge on the basic physiology of the process from which many principles of management become self-evident;

or a combination of these.

There are four overriding clinical messages:

1. A sound knowledge of the physiology of suckling, milk transfer and the determinants of milk quality is essential to resolving apparent problems of breast milk insufficiency.
2. Only a tiny proportion of women are unable to produce sufficient milk to meet their baby's needs.
3. The vast majority of apparent problems can be overcome by referring the mother to someone with specialist skills and ability in managing breast feeding.
4. Mothers benefit most from support and reassurance from professional staff.

Paediatricians, in common with all health care workers, must develop confidence that the basic mechanisms of breast feeding will work for women. This is essential to ensure that women's own self confidence in their ability to breast feed is not undermined.

References

1. Standing Committee on Nutrition of the British Paediatric Association. Is breast feeding beneficial in the UK? *Archives of Disease in Childhood* 1994; **71**: 376–80
2. White A, Freeth S, O'Brien M. *Infant feeding 1990.* London: HMSO, Office of Population Censuses and Surveys, 1992
3. Prentice AM, Goldberg GR, Prentice A. Body mass index and lactation performance. *European Journal of Clinical Nutrition* 1994; **48**(Suppl 3): S78–89

4. Dugdale AE. Evolution and infant feeding. *Lancet* 1986; **i**: 670–3
5. Prentice AM, Paul AA, Prentice A, Black AE, *et al.* Cross-cultural differences in lactational performance. In: Hamosh M, Goldman AS, eds. *Human lactation 2.* New York: Plenum Press, 1986: 13–44
6. Jackson DA, Imong SM, Silprasert A, Ruckphaopunt S, *et al.* Circadian variation in fat concentration of breast-milk in a rural northern Thai population. *British Journal of Nutrition* 1988; **59**: 349–63
7. Neville MC. Regulation of mammary development and lactation. In: Neville MC, Neifert MR, eds. *Lactation: physiology, nutrition, and breast-feeding.* New York: Plenum Press, 1983
8. Neville MC, Keller R, Seacat J, Lutes V, *et al.* Studies in human lactation; milk volumes in lactating women during the onset of lactation and full lactation. *American Journal of Clinical Nutrition* 1988; **48**: 1375–86
9. Drewett K, Amatayakul K, Wongsawasdii L, Mangklabruks A, *et al.* Nursing frequency and the energy intake from breast milk and supplementary food in a rural Thai population: a longitudinal study. *European Journal of Clinical Nutrition* 1993; **47**: 880–91
10. Stuff J, Nichols B. Nutrient intake and growth performance in older infants fed human milk. *Journal of Pediatrics* 1989; **115**: 959–68
11. Karlberg J. *Modelling of human growth.* Göteborg, Sweden, 1987
12. Whitehead RG. Infant physiology, nutritional requirements, and lactational adequacy. *American Journal of Clinical Nutrition* 1985; **41**: 447–58
13. Peaker M, Wilde CJ. Evidence for local feedback control of human milk secretion. *News in Physiological Science* 1987; **2**: 124–6
14. Prentice A, Addey CV, Wilde CJ. Evidence for local feedback control of human milk secretion. *Biochemical Society Transactions* 1989; **17**: 489–92
15. Daly SE, Kent JC, Huynh Du Q, Owens RA, *et al.* The determination of short-term breast volume changes and the rate of synthesis of human milk using computerized breast measurement. *Experimental Physiology* 1992; **77**: 79–87
16. Dewey KG, Heining J, Nommsen LA, Lonnerdal B. Maternal versus infant factors related to breast milk intake and residual milk volume: the DARLING study. *Pediatrics* 1991; **87**: 829–37
17. Woolridge MW, Baum JD. Infant appetite-control and the regulation of breast milk supply. *Children's Hospital Quarterly* 1991; **3**: 113–9
18. Fomon SJ, Filler LJ, Thomas LN, Anderson TA, Nelson SE. Influence of formula concentration on caloric intake and growth of normal infants. *Acta Paediatrica Scandinavica* 1975; **75**: 893–8
19. Woolridge MW, Ingram JC, Baum JD. Do changes in pattern of breast usage alter the baby's nutrient intake? *Lancet* 1990; **336**: 395–7
20. Drewett RF, Woolridge MW, Greasley V, McLeod CN, *et al.* Evaluating breast-milk intake by test weighing: a portable electronic balance suitable for community and field studies. *Early Human Development* 1984; **10**: 123–6
21. Davies DP. Is inadequate breast feeding an important cause of failure to thrive? *Lancet* 1979; **i**: 541–2

3 | Food for the weanling: have we improved?

Brian Wharton
Director-General, British Nutrition Foundation, London

Jane Morgan
Senior Lecturer in Nutrition, University of Surrey

At a conference on food for the weanling in 1986, Wharton commented:

> The 1970s was the decade of the suckling and the priority for the 1980s should have been the weanling. Halfway through the decade we have failed to grasp the weanling's nettle.[1]

Some eight years later, and well into the next decade, have we improved? The answer is yes but we could do better.

The sources of evidence

We are fortunate in Britain in having a series of data produced for the ministries and government departments which give an overall nutritional view of changes in nutritional opinion and practice. The first in the series of reports on present-day practice in infant feeding was produced in 1974.[2] Since then there have been two further reports in this series,[3,4] together with two associated reports, *Composition of human milk*[5] and *Artificial feeds for the young infant*.[6] Recently, a further report dealing specifically with weaning and the weaning diet has been published.[7]

What has been happening in infant feeding since 1975 is recorded in the quinquennial reports on infant feeding prepared by the Office of Population Censuses and Surveys.[8–11] Earlier versions concentrated on breast feeding with limited other information, but the more recent reports provide more information. Finally, the Ministry of Agriculture, Fisheries and Food (MAFF) has published the results of a 1984 survey on the diets of older infants (6–12 months old).[12]

There have also been a number of local surveys, particularly in inner-city areas. A European Union committee has given recommendations concerning the composition of weaning foods,[13] which might eventually pass into European law.[14]

As the child crosses the weanling's bridge[1] he continues to receive the suckling's foods, begins to receive special weaning foods, either commercially available or prepared by his mother, and finally family foods are introduced. These will be considered in turn.

The suckling's food

Table 1 shows the prevalence of breast feeding from four months of age onwards. Between 1975 and 1980 there was a welcome increase in the percentage of babies breast fed at four months but there has been little change since then. Most mothers breast feeding at four months continued until six months. If the aim is to increase the number of breast fed babies in the early months of weaning, the influence must be effected earlier—it seems that mothers still breast feeding at four months are sufficiently motivated to continue for some time.

The infant formulas and milks received in later infancy in recent years are shown in Table 2. The secular comparisons indicate two trends. First, there has been a welcome decrease in the number receiving unmodified whole cow's milk. There is, however, a long way to go—42% were still receiving unmodified cow's milk instead of an infant formula or follow-on milk at the age of nine months. Second, the choice of infant formula has changed, more now favouring a casein-predominant formula rather than a whey-based one. There is no good reason for this change but it is probably harmless. A belief exists in Britain, but in no other country, that casein formulas are more satisfying—despite double-blind trials

Table 1. Percentage of breast feeding from the age of four months (England and Wales) (from Refs 8–11)

Year	4 months (%)	6 months (%)	9 months (%)
1975	15	10	<5
1980	27	23	12
1985	26	21	11
1990	25	21	12

Table 2. Liquid part of diet received by bottle fed babies (Great Britain) (from Refs 10 & 11)

Milk/infant formula	4–5 months (%)		9–10 months (%)	
	1985	1990	1985	1990
Whey	43	32	12	18
Casein	46	61	16	33
Other	4	4	4	7
Cow's milk	7	3	67	42

showing little difference in mothers' appreciation of satiety in their babies receiving the two types of formula.

Comparison of the breast and bottle feeding groups showed that more breast fed babies receive unmodified cow's milk as a bottle feed. Perhaps breast feeding mothers find the inconvenience of making up a bottle feed from powdered formula for a top-up is too great. The problem for these babies is that they receive little iron from the liquid parts of their diet (whether breast milk or unmodified cow's milk), so a good source of available iron is essential in the rest of the weanling's diet—but do they receive it?

Time of weaning

There was also a substantial change in the age of introduction of solid food between 1975 and 1980 but little change since then (Table 3). Nevertheless, the majority of mothers ignore the current

Table 3. Percentage of infants given solid food at different ages (from Refs 8–11)

Year	6 weeks (%)	3 months (%)	4 months (%)
1975 (England & Wales)	40	85	97
1980 (Great Britain)	14	52	89
1985 (Great Britain)	11	62	90
1990 (Great Britain)	9	68	94

advice to delay weaning until 3–4 months. The oft-quoted 4–6 months of age dates from the original report of the Department of Health[2] which has been widely adopted (eg by the World Health Organisation (WHO), the American Academy of Pediatrics and, more recently, again in Britain[7]). This choice of age is based more on experienced opinion than on hard scientific analysis. Now that young infants receive breast milk or a modern infant formula rather than the higher protein, high sodium, higher renal solute load cow's milk, and manufactured weaning foods contain less protein, less salt and are often gluten-free, the timing may not be so critical.

A recent survey in Dundee[15] has not detected any adverse effects in babies who are weaned earlier, so perhaps mothers are right in their flexible approach to the age of weaning. Many mothers are advised to introduce solid foods earlier than three months by members of the primary health care team, particularly health visitors. Certainly it seems that views of 'expert committees' do not reach the grass-roots health care professionals. One initiative of *The health of the nation*[16] is to improve the nutritional knowledge of these groups.

Weaning foods and family foods

The mean energy and nutrient contents of savoury and sweet home-prepared weaning meals for infants aged 3–11 months are listed in Table 4 and compared with the current European Commission (EC) draft directive on the nutrient composition of weaning foods commercially available.[14] Some of the home-prepared meals contain more fat and more carbohydrate, and many contain more sodium, than the EC draft directive recommends; about 40% of the meals had an energy content less than that of human milk.[17] Thus, they often do not conform to the conventional wisdom that home-prepared weaning meals are nutritionally superior to commercially available ones. The study by MAFF[12] found that infants aged 6–9 months fed predominantly commercial weaning foods received, on average, less protein, fat, fibre and sugar each day, and more iron and vitamin D, than those receiving family foods. As family foods are introduced, it seems some care is necessary to maintain a healthy diet.

Minerals

Iron deficiency anaemia is still with us. It is common in Britain, but almost unknown in Hong Kong—we have no room for complacency

Table 4. Energy and nutrient contents (mean and standard deviation) of savoury and sweet home-prepared weaning foods compared with those recommended in the draft European Commission (EC) directive.[14]

	Draft EC directive	Home-prepared savoury (SD)	Not meeting draft EC directive (%)	Home-prepared sweet (SD)	Not meeting draft EC directive (%)
Energy (kcal/100 g)		89 (44)	N/A	87 (33)	N/A
Fat (g/100 kcal)	≯6 g/100 kcal where meat or cheese main ingredient	2.4 (1.7)	2	N/A	N/A
	≯4.5 g/100 kcal for all other savoury products	2.4 (1.7)	14	N/A	N/A
Protein (g/100 kcal)	≮3 g/100 kcal	6.0 (3.0)	12	N/A	N/A
Carbohydrate (g/100 g)	≯20 g/100 g for pure fruit desserts	N/A	N/A	13.5 (4.6)	7
	≯25 g/100 g for other desserts and puddings	N/A	N/A	14.5 (6.2)	4
Sodium (mg/100 kcal)	≯200 mg/100 kcal	153.7 (144.6)	31	49.7 (53.1)	3
Iron (mg/100 g)		0.9 (0.6)	N/A	0.4 (0.3)	N/A
Zinc (mg/100 g)		0.8 (0.8)	N/A	0.4 (0.3)	N/A

N/A = no appropriate draft EC directive.

(see Table 5). The only explanation for this difference appears to be the extended use in Hong Kong of iron-fortified infant formulas throughout infancy and into the second year of life.

Clearly, it is possible to design diets which contain whole cow's milk as the main drink but which also provide a satisfactory amount of absorbable haem iron (eg from meat), but most studies of actual practice show that the use of iron-fortified formulas throughout

Table 5. Percentage of infants with anaemia or low ferritin in the United Kingdom (nationally representative sample)[7] and Hong Kong (Shatin area)[18]

Age (months)	Number	Anaemia (Hb <11 g/dl) (%)	Low ferritin (mcg/1) (%)
United Kingdom			
18–29	300	12	<10: 28
30–41	353	6	<10: 18
Hong Kong			
18	150	2	<7: 1

infancy rather than the earlier introduction of unmodified cow's milk is associated with a better iron status.

The daily intake of nutrients from all sources in older infants (6–12 months) grouped according to the main milk consumed is shown in Table 6. Those consuming an infant formula received more appropriate amounts of protein (less) and iron (more) than those receiving only whole cow's milk. The same study showed that infants aged 6–9 months fed predominantly commercial infant foods had an average iron intake of 10 mg compared to 5 mg in those receiving mainly family foods in the solid part of their diet.[12]

There is no overt evidence of zinc deficiency in this country, but there are some concerns in both the developed and the developing worlds (see Table 7). There should perhaps be a more concentrated effort to assess zinc nutritional status in British children: the problem is twofold, in that 'tests' of zinc nutrition are difficult to interpret and the 'gold standard' for demonstrating deficiency is still the effects of zinc supplementation.

Since breast milk contains only small amounts of iron and the concentration of zinc falls with increasing length of lactation, it has been argued that the best weaning food for breast fed babies is meat in order to supply these two minerals. Bottle fed babies receive adequate amounts of iron and zinc from infant formula, so other weaning foods such as cereals are satisfactory.

Vitamins

Vitamin D deficiency rickets is now less common—at least, that is most people's impression, but hard figures are not available. Assuming the assumption is correct, it is not clear why the prevalence has

Table 6. Daily intake of nutrients from all sources (both liquid and solid foods) of infants aged 6–12 months grouped according to main milk consumed (modified from Ref. 12)

Nutrient	Breast* milk (n = 48)	Infant formula (n = 267)	Cow's milk (n = 150)	RNI for 7–9 months
Protein (g)	21.0	26.2	34.8	13.7
Fat (g)	30.9	35.3	37.5	
Calcium (mg)	512	689	880	525
Iron (mg)	6.4	11.3	6.7	7.8
Zinc (mg)	3.6	4.5	4.7	5.0
Retinol (µg)	519	801	462	350
Carotene (µg)	844	961	1250	
Vitamin D (µg)	1.0	9.1	1.0	7
Vitamin C (mg)	76	135	85	25
Energy (kcal)	718	871	901	800

*Note small number; they were younger and therefore smaller than the other two groups.
RNI = reference nutrient intake (estimated average requirement for energy).

Table 7. Possible reasons for concern about zinc nutrition

● Growth faltering in:
  — breast fed immigrant children in France
  — immigrant toddlers in Denver, Colorado, USA

● Absorption affected by iron and soya in formulas

● Low median dietary intake by British weanlings

● Impaired growth during treatment for kwashiorkor in Jamaica

● Delayed puberty in Iran

decreased because there is less use today of vitamin supplements.[11] Perhaps the vitamin D status of mothers has improved, so that their children have better stores at birth. Even supposing this speculation is correct, what is the reason? The infant's longer use of an infant formula (all of which are fortified with vitamin D in Britain) may well be responsible. The Clean Air Act may also have played a role in improving the status of mothers and their babies.

There seems no reason to be concerned about the possibility of other vitamin deficiencies in British weanlings. In the developing world, vitamin A deficiency has long received considerable attention as a cause of xerophthalmia, keratomalacia and eventually blindness. More recently, however, there has been mounting evidence from several countries in the developing world that vitamin A supplements, even in the absence of clinically overt deficiency, reduce child mortality (see Table 8). Does this also have some message for developed countries? Are there pockets of vitamin A deficiency in underprivileged groups in this country? All that can be said at present is that there is no evidence to support this suggestion.

Patients or products

A problem with nutrition is how easily a single nutrient, a single product or a single technique can dominate our approach. For example, the problems of iron may be stressed. Some groups see breast milk as the answer to everything, others promote their follow-on formula, yet others defend the place of cow's milk. Weaning shows how important it is to have a patient (or client or consumer) orientated approach, not a product orientated one. Breast milk promotion organisations, infant food manufacturers and the dairy industry might take a service industry as their model rather than a product one. 'Man shall not live by bread alone', nor at this age by breast milk alone, follow-on milk alone or cow's milk alone—a portfolio of appropriately used foods should be promoted.

A final point concerns the role of nutrition in the overall growth and development of the child. While some problems can be analysed in clear terms of primary nutrient deficiency or excess, in other instances the disturbed nutrition is just one more factor in, or one more symptom of, a mother and child relationship which is under stress, for whatever intrinsic or environmental cause.

Verdict

By 1986, the weanling's lot had already improved from that described in the 1974 report:[2] weaning was later, coeliac disease and very rapid weight gains were both less common. Since then rickets has (probably) come under control, but there is still a substantial amount of iron deficiency. Should we not be ashamed that our

Table 8. Child mortality and vitamin A supplementation

Place	Dose (1,000 units)	Dosing frequency	Reduction in deaths (%)
Tamil Nadu	8.3	weekly	54
Hyderabad	200	6 monthly	—
Nepal	200	4 monthly	30
Sudan	200	6 monthly	—
Indonesia	200	6 monthly	34
Ghana	200	4 monthly	19

weanlings fare worse in this respect than in some other countries such as Hong Kong?

What should be the strategy for prevention? One approach is to screen for anaemia, with early detection and treatment. Fiscal measures such as the provision of subsidised fortified foods play a small role in this country under the family support provisions and a much bigger one in countries such as the USA and Chile. Fortification of infant foods means that all infants receiving them consume extra amounts of iron whether or not they need it, and irrespective of their iron status. In principle, this approach, targeted only by age and not necessarily by need, is undesirable. Nevertheless, it seems to be effective. If fortified foods are to be effective, however, a mother must be prepared to use commercially available foods—and some frown on this. But why? Of course, preparing her baby's food is one of the mother's expressions of love, but there seems no reason why she should not make sensible use of the milk products (infant formulas and follow-on milks) and weaning foods specifically designed for this age group.

References

1. Wharton BA. Food for the weanling: the next priority in infant nutrition. *Acta Paediatrica Scandinavica* 1986; **323** (Suppl): 96–102
2. Department of Health and Social Security. *Present-day practice in infant feeding.* Report on health and social subjects no. 9. London: HMSO, 1974
3. Department of Health and Social Security. *Present-day practice in infant feeding. 1980.* Report on health and social subjects no. 20. London: HMSO, 1980

4. Department of Health and Social Security. *Present-day practice in infant feeding: third report.* Report on health and social subjects no. 32. London: HMSO, 1988

5. Department of Health and Social Security. *Composition of human milk.* Report on health and social subjects no. 12. London: HMSO, 1977

6. Department of Health and Social Security. *Artificial feeds for the young infant.* Report on health and social subjects no. 18. London: HMSO, 1980

7. Department of Health. *Weaning and the weaning diet.* Report on health and social subjects no. 45. London: HMSO, 1994

8. Martin J. *Infant feeding 1975: attitudes and practice in England and Wales.* London: HMSO, 1978

9. Martin J, Monk S. *Infant feeding 1980.* London: Office of Population Censuses and Surveys, 1982

10. Martin J, White A. *Infant feeding 1985.* London: HMSO, 1988

11. White A, Freeth S, O'Brien M. *Infant feeding 1990.* London: HMSO, 1992

12. Mills A, Tyler H. *Food and nutrient intakes of British infants aged 6–12 months.* London: HMSO, 1992

13. Commission of the European Communities. *First report on the essential requirements for weaning foods.* Reports of the Scientific Committee for Food, 24th series, no. EUR 13140-EN. Luxembourg: Office for official publications of the European Communities, 1991

14. *Processed cereal-based foods and baby foods for infants and young children.* Draft Commission directive III/5886/94-EN. Brussels: European Commission, US/UNIC1/04/03/00/BM/dm, 1993

15. Forsyth SJ, Ogston SA, Clark A, Florey C du V, Howie PW. Relationship between early introduction of solid food to infants and their weight and illnesses during the first two years of life. *British Medical Journal* 1993; **306**: 1572–6

16. Department of Health. *The health of the nation—a strategy for health in England.* London: HMSO, 1992

17. Stordy BJ, Redfern AM, Morgan JB. Healthy eating for infants—mothers' actions. *Acta Paediatrica Scandinavica* 1995 (in press)

18. Leung SSF, Davies DP, Lui S, Lo L, *et al.* Iron deficiency is uncommon in healthy Hong Kong infants at 18 months. *Journal of Tropical Pediatrics* 1988; **34**: 100–3

4 | Nutrition in the normal infant: opportunities in primary care

John James
General Practitioner, Montpelier Health Centre, Bristol

Nutrition in infancy is a major determinant of growth and development, and exerts considerable influence on adult health. The field of infant nutrition is attracting considerable research interest, and public awareness of the importance of early nutrition has never been greater. Unfortunately, there are few clear guidelines on healthy nutrition for infants, in part because of the difficulty in interpreting the research findings.[1] The 1994 Committee on Medical Aspects of Food Policy (COMA) report, *Weaning and the weaning diet,*[2] is, however, both timely and welcome. It is beyond dispute, though, that the primary care team is ideally placed to influence the dietary habits of parents and their children.

This chapter will consider the positive developments in primary care which offer exciting opportunities for improving childhood nutrition in the community, and describe the dietary interventions that have been introduced in my own practice. I will suggest that there is considerable opportunity for nutrition research in primary care which, in combination with clear nutritional guidelines, education for the primary care team, and targeted, community based interventions, could form the basis of a strategy for the future.

Childhood nutrition education in the community today

The influence of nutrition on child development and its impact on adult life is beyond the scope of this chapter. However, the epidemiological studies of Barker and co-workers[3] linking low birth weight and underweight at one year with increased risk of cardiovascular disease in adulthood have attracted considerable interest, and received extensive coverage in the media. As a result, there is increased public interest and awareness of the importance of healthy nutrition. Families expect primary care workers to provide advice about healthy nutrition, and nutritional advice is regarded as a priority. A survey of 300 mothers (SMA nutrition market research, 1991) showed that 94% expected clear guidelines about a weaning diet, and felt that health visitors and general practitioners (GPs) should offer advice automatically. Only 25% of the mothers had received weaning advice; more than half found the advice confusing or unhelpful. In 1992, in my own inner city practice in a deprived part of Bristol, 100 mothers were asked about their own and their children's health needs. A majority identified nutrition advice as the most important need. These and other surveys support the need for the primary care team to take an active role in providing nutritional advice for young children.

Positive developments in primary care paediatrics

Child care services offered by GPs are developing rapidly. There has been a shift away from the purely 'reactive' services for children and their carers towards more preventive and anticipatory services. There is a welcome move towards team-work, with GPs beginning to recognise that other members of the primary care team have skills that are often more appropriate than their own to the needs of families. Now that they have taken responsibility for child health surveillance, GPs are also recognising the importance of the input from health visitors. A symbiosis is developing.

Furthermore, the majority of doctors entering general practice today will have had experience of hospital paediatrics, and an increasing number will also have had training in community paediatrics. As a result, practices will be offering a wider range of services for children and their families, with orientation towards preventive services. Community paediatricians now work closely with practices, and many have set up secondary clinics in health centres.

There is increased recognition that parents are the principal carers for their children and are concerned for their well-being. Parents are extremely receptive to advice regarding a healthy lifestyle for their children, and are likely to heed the advice given.

The *Health of the Nation* targets,[4] and the emphasis placed on a healthy lifestyle as a key component of general practice services (with considerable financial implications to participating practices), have resulted in practices focusing more on health promotion. Effective health promotion depends on team-work, so team building in practices has developed considerably. Many practices have found the experience enjoyable.

The majority of practices are now computerised and use sophisticated databases. Initially introduced to help with practice management, their use enables all aspects of patient care to be monitored. Health promotion details are also recorded and monitored and, increasingly, social background, medical and health behaviour details. With standardisation of data collection (Reed codes are already installed on all practice computer systems), this may prove to be a powerful tool for research.

Nutritional interventions in Montpelier Health Centre

Montpelier Health Centre is an inner city practice characterised by severe socio-economic deprivation. Mothers struggle to bring up their children against a background of poverty, poor housing (10% are homeless), violence and drug abuse:

- 70% of the mothers are unsupported;
- 25% of the mothers are under 20 years old;
- 45% are Afro-Caribbean;
- 950 children under the age of five are registered with the practice; and
- nearly 100 are on the child protection register.

The practice is committed to close team-work, and some modest successes in improving nutrition have been recorded.

Rickets in Rastafarian children

As a result of two children presenting in 1985 with nutritional rickets, 48 children under two years whose parents adhered to a strict vegan diet prescribed by their Rastafarian beliefs were screened. They were identified from the computerised age-sex register by a Rastafarian mother. All the children were X-rayed and had blood estimation for alkaline phosphate and haemoglobin.

Seven children were found to have nutritional rickets, and 14 iron deficiency anaemia (IDA).[5] By involving a local community leader who endorsed (on local television) the use of vitamin D, the condition was treated, dietary information was given to all mothers, and no further cases have been found. This demonstrated that, by approaching the problem sensitively and offering mothers an acceptable form of prevention and treatment, an important nutritional deficiency can be treated and prevented.

Iron deficiency anaemia

IDA is the leading cause of anaemia in children in the UK and the commonest nutritional disorder during weaning. It is related to poverty and ethnic minority status, with a prevalence of up to 28% in at-risk populations in the second year of life. Psychomotor delay and behavioural disorder are serious consequences,[6] which are potentially reversible although they may persist long-term.[7]

In 1986 it was therefore decided to investigate the feasibility of screening children in our practice for IDA. A total of 521 children aged between one and five years were invited to attend for capillary estimation of haemoglobin. It was found that 21.9% of the 365 (70%) children who responded, 35.8% of the one year olds and 45.8% of the Afro-Caribbean children in this age group were anaemic (haemoglobin <115 g/l). As a result, screening for IDA was introduced for all children when attending for measles/MMR immunisation at 14 months. At the same time, a programme of dietary education for mothers was introduced by midwives antenatally, and by health visitors and doctors in the first year of life. The importance was emphasised of fortified formula milks and weaning foods rich in iron. A year later, only 23.7% of 122 children screened at 14 months (coverage 96%) were anaemic.[8]

It was disappointing to find that by 1990 the prevalence of IDA had risen to 34.2%; this probably related to less emphasis being placed on dietary education subsequent to an impressive reduction in IDA achieved the previous year. Subsequent follow-up has shown an annual prevalence of around 22%, emphasising the importance of continuing both dietary education and audit.

In order to investigate further the natural history of IDA, 150 children who were screened at 14 months were followed up a year later. The results demonstrated a complex relationship between haemoglobin at 14 months and 2 years, but the earlier value was not predictive of the latter; children whose weight was below the tenth centile or who were difficult to feed in the second year of life were at increased risk of anaemia.[9] These results suggest that screening alone is unlikely to prevent the adverse effects of IDA.

Improving the diet of young mothers and their children

Encouraged by mothers' expressed need for nutritional advice (see above), the health visitors introduced a programme of dietary education for young mothers.[10] They identified 44 young mothers who were seen to be struggling with their own and their children's diets. All were willing to take part in the programme, which involved one-to-one teaching with their own health visitor. The programme was devised with the help of the dietitians who supervised a number of seminars for practice staff. A list of desirable food groups was established, as well as aspects of organisation and planning (Table 1).

This list was scored using specially devised dietary diaries (each 'desirable' food attracting one point), and could be used as a syllabus for teaching. Mothers received between six and ten one-to-one teaching sessions in their homes, and the diaries were rescored. Scores improved from 6.7 (out of a possible 15) to 10.2. Successful introductions to the children's diets are shown (Table 2). Mothers said that they enjoyed the project, and most of them felt that their children's diet had improved; overall, improved levels of self esteem were demonstrated in these mothers.

Table 1. Food choices and organisation of meals.

Desirable food choices
- one protein food
- another protein food
- protein containing iron
- potatoes, pasta, rice
- one fruit portion, juice
- another fruit portion, juice
- one serving of vegetables (not potatoes)
- bread
- another high fibre food
- half pint full cream milk for child
- half pint milk for mother

Organisation and planning
- plan meal in advance
- eat meals together
- regular meals

Table 2. Breakdown of children's diets.

Commonly absent	Successfully introduced
Milk	Yes
Fruit	Yes
Another fruit	No
Protein containing iron	Yes
Two servings of vegetables	No
Eating meals together	Yes
Regular meals	Yes

Following the success of this intervention, a number of mothers proposed that the project be continued—but in a group setting. To date, 86 mothers have formed 23 groups who meet, plan a meal, shop, cook and eat together on a regular basis. Health visitors supervise the groups when asked, and we have been able to pay for the food. As before, dietary scores have improved significantly.

Thus, even in conditions of deprivation (when food costs have been shown to be a barrier to purchasing healthy foods) it is possible to improve both the children's diet and the mothers' feeling of well-being.

A strategy for the future

If the primary care team is to improve child nutrition, there is a need for clear nutritional guidelines. The recently published COMA report on weaning diet[2] will pave the way for the development of weaning protocols that should impact on infants. As indicated above, information must be appropriate to the levels of knowledge, culture and expectations of practice populations. Local community paediatricians should take a lead in developing local protocols. I hope that further guidelines will follow.

Nutrition is afforded little space in medical syllabuses, and there is a real need for programmes of dietary education for primary care teams. As well as covering basic nutrition facts, courses should cover aspects of health promotion and develop teaching skills. There should be an opportunity to cover specific needs of practice populations (eg the diet of families of minority ethnic groups).

Targeted interventions can be effective and rewarding for primary care teams. Our screening programme for IDA has proved effective and worthwhile, and is now being introduced to other inner city practices in Bristol as well as community child health clinics in Lambeth, South London. Community paediatricians are well placed to introduce other appropriate programmes into primary care. Properly funded, they may prove popular with primary care teams.

There are many opportunities for research in primary care. For example, the COMA weaning diet panel identified a number of questions relating to IDA:

- the feasibility of screening for IDA;
- the feasibility of prevention of IDA through dietary advice; and
- the natural history of the condition.

Our studies on IDA provide some of the answers but larger scale investigations are indicated. Properly co-ordinated, and using the database which is now held by most general practitioners, these and other important questions may be answered. Community based nutrition interventions are under-researched, yet have considerable potential to influence healthy nutrition. These opportunities must not be missed.

Conclusion

Child nutrition has a major influence on child development and later life. With increased public awareness of the importance of diet, the primary care team, with increasing skills in paediatrics and health promotion, is ideally placed to improve the nutrition of children today.

References

1. Lucas A. Role of nutritional programming in determining adult morbidity. *Archives of Disease in Childhood* 1994; **71**: 288–90
2. Department of Health report on health and social subjects. Committee on Medical Aspects of Food Policy. *Weaning and the weaning diet.* Report of the working group on the weaning diet. London: Department of Health, 1994
3. Barker DJP, Meade TW, Fall CHD, Lee A, *et al.* Relation of fetal and infant growth to plasma fibrinogen and factor VII concentrations in adult life. *British Medical Journal.* 1992; **304**: 148–52
4. Department of Health. *The health of the nation—a strategy for health in England.* London: HMSO, 1992
5. James JA, Clark C, Ward PS. Screening Rastafarian children for nutritional rickets. *British Medical Journal* 1992; **304**: 376–8
6. Oski FA. Iron deficiency anemia in infancy and childhood. *New England Journal of Medicine* 1993; **329**: 190–3
7. Lozoff B, Jiminez E, Wolf AW. Long term development outcome of infants with iron deficiency. *New England Journal of Medicine* 1992; **325**: 687–94
8. James JA, Lawson P, Male P, Oakhill A. Preventing iron deficiency anaemia in pre-school children by implementing an educational and screening programme in an inner city practice. *British Medical Journal* 1989; **299**: 838–40
9. James J, Laing G, Logan S. Screening for iron deficiency anaemia in primary care. *British Medical Journal* 1995 (in press)
10. James J, Brown J, Douglas M, Cox J, Stocker S. Improving the diet of under fives in a deprived inner city practice. *Health Trends* 1992; **24**: 161–4

PART TWO

Nutrition in neonatal care

5 | Human milk: a sacred cow? A quest for optimum nutrition for pre-term babies

D P Davies
Professor and Head of the University Department of Child Health, University of Wales College of Medicine, Cardiff

> One of the most important side-effects of a breast milk bank is that it stimulates doctors, nurses and others to interest themselves in the physiology and importance of breast feeding.[1]

We hardly need to be reminded of the dramatic improvements in the survival of prematurely born babies in recent years brought about by the many advances in perinatal care over this period. Successful management of early cardiorespiratory hazards (the major contributor to early death), however, brings with it all too often one very real problem that has its origins in the physiologically unprepared state of the gastrointestinal tract and metabolism of these small babies to digest, absorb and utilise nutrients: how are they to be optimally nourished when, without premature birth, they would have been fed across the placenta with a physiological blend of nutrients prepared by the mother? Many of these small babies will be sick or extremely immature and need an initial period of parenteral feeding but, in time, enteral nutrition has to be established in those who survive. What is the best nutrition for them?

Optimum nutrition for pre-term babies

Optimum nutrition for pre-term babies is that which permits, in the short-term, satisfactory growth and health free from metabolic problems and infection, and in the long-term fulfilment of genetically endowed growth and psychomotor potential and physical well-being. For babies born at term there can be no doubt of the superiority of human milk to provide these needs, above all else because of the high digestibility of its fat, readily utilisable nitrogen, long-chain polyunsaturated fatty acids for optimum biomembrane synthesis, an appropriate balance of minerals and electrolytes, and an antimicrobial umbrella of immune substances which offers

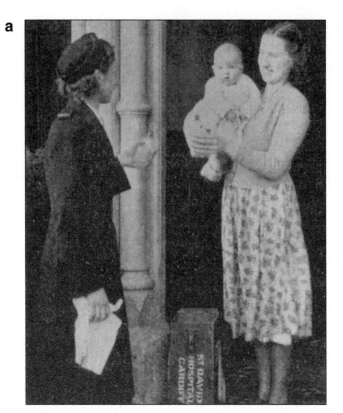

Fig 1. *Scenes from the milk bank at St David's Hospital, Cardiff, in the early 1950s.* **a**: doorstep collection; **b**: pooling the milk; **c**: pasteurisation and storage.

protection against infections, especially of the gastrointestinal tract. This assumption of the biological superiority of human milk was also held for a long time as a tenet of faith for pre-term babies. In the early part of this century it motivated the setting up, in maternity hospitals in economically developed countries, of human milk banks with responsibilities to collect, process, store and administer human milk to babies whose mothers were unable to provide enough of their own milk. For these babies, milk was provided by other breast-feeding mothers, and came to be termed donor breast milk (Figure 1).

Emerging doubts over the nutritional suitability of human milk

All seemed well until the 1970s when doubts arose about the suitability of donor breast milk for babies born prematurely. Studies revealed:

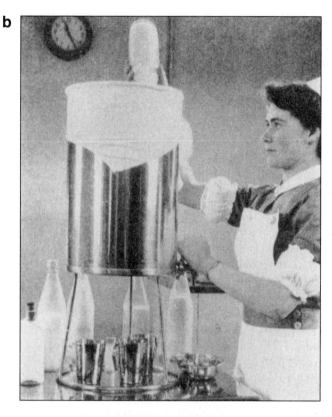

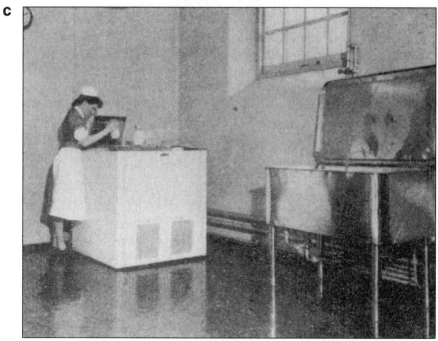

- this milk to be nutritionally heterogeneous and often of poor quality;[2]
- slower growth rates in babies fed human milk;[3]
- questionable antimicrobial benefits because the heat applied to donor milk to free it of microbial contamination was found to destroy many of the physiological functions of its specific antimicrobial properties.[4]

A sacred cow had begun its demise, poignantly described by Dr Herbert Barrie in his reference to the milk bank in St David's Hospital, Cardiff:

> Thirty years ago, the milk came frozen on the night train from Cardiff, and was collected by nurses in the bleak and chilly dawn on Paddington Station. Back at the ranch, from Llandough to Llanedeyrn, the mothers took their milk to St David's at a penny an ounce to feed premature babies in London and make ends meet at home. Quality checks were unheard of but if it passed the sharp eyes and nose of the bank sister, with a fearsome reputation for sniffing out the merest drop of added water, it was widely regarded the ideal food for premature babies. The results were not good and said more for the fortitude of babies than the milk squirted into their mouths through Belcroy feeders. But with a perinatal mortality of 35 per cent and wages under the breadline, a milk bank only had beggars, not choosers.[5]

These anxieties were not new. Confidence in human milk as the ideal food for pre-term babies had been challenged as early as 1919 by Finkelstein in Germany;[6] thereafter, doubts had been repeatedly expressed that human milk might not offer the best nutrition for babies born very early in the third trimester with their special nutrition and growth requirements.[7,8] However, these voices were lone cries. The notion of the uniqueness of breast milk generally continued to reign supreme.

It is worth examining some of these doubts about the nutritional suitability of human milk in a little more detail in order to understand future events.

Poor milk quality

Breast milk given to these small infants was usually a 'cocktail' of various milks depending upon methods of collection.

Mature expressed milk was obtained from the breast by hand expression or by electric hand pump after a feed by a mother well established in breast feeding her own normal baby—a method of collection widely used in traditional human milk banks.

Table 1. Average composition of pooled expressed and drip milk (taken from Gibbs *et al.*[2])

Milk component	Expressed	Drip
Energy (kcal/l)	700	480
Protein (g/l)	10.7	100
Lactose (g/l)	74	65
Fat (g/l)	42	22
Sodium (mmol/l)	6.4	5.5
Potassium (mmol/l)	15	16.1
Calcium (mmol/l)	8.7	6.9
Magnesium (mmol/l)	1.2	1.2

Drip milk 'dripped' passively and was collected from the non-feeding breast during a feed. It was this practice that came under increasing scrutiny in the 1970s, chiefly because the milk was found to contain much less fat, and therefore energy, than expressed milk (on average, 480 cal/l and 700 cal/l, respectively)[2,9] (Table 1)—an effect accentuated even more by the natural fall in fat content with time post-partum.

Combined drip and expressed milk was collected to provide a food with advantages over drip or expressed milk alone. A greater volume could be obtained and the energy content was only slightly less than that of expressed milk.[10]

Pre-term milk came to be the term used for the small amount of milk which mothers giving birth prematurely could express themselves. Its composition was to capture clinical interest only in the 1970s, paralleling the general reawakening of interest in breast feeding at this time. Before this, little attempt was made to encourage these mothers to breast feed so its composition was not seen to deserve detailed analysis. Pre-term milk was found to contain:

- about 20% more nitrogen, including non-protein nitrogen;[11]
- secretory immunoglobulin (Ig) A;[12]
- more cholesterol, phospholipids and long-chain polyunsaturated fatty acids (the biomembrane substrates of milk);[13] and
- higher concentrations of sodium and chloride, but less calcium and phosphate.[14]

The overall composition of pre-term milk was typical of a prolonged colostral phase.

This nutritional variability in milk given to the baby was compounded by other influences during its preparation and administration. Williamson and colleagues found that fat absorption after pasteurisation was only 73% that of unheated milk,[15] most likely due to the destruction of breast milk bile salt stimulated lipase. Protein utilisation was also adversely affected by heat.[15] During feeding, fat was often left sticking to the walls of the delivery tubes, syringe pumps and burettes used in administering milk; up to 35% of the milk energy content could be lost in this way.[16,17] Nutritional proteins and immunoglobulins were also lost in the process.

These variations in important milk nutrients were unacceptable to many clinicians and weakened the argument to continue to feed human milk to pre-term infants.

Poor growth and its consequences

Doubts had been repeatedly expressed since early this century that growth rates of pre-term babies were less than would be expected in the normally growing fetus at an equivalent stage of development.[6-8] The 1970s were to see a rebirth of this concern, and there emerged little doubt that pre-term babies fed whatever type or combination of human milk grew less well in weight, length and head circumference than those fed milk formula—both conventional and special low birth weight milks.[3] A good illustration of this was provided by Lucas et al who showed that a 1.2 kg baby fed donor human milk would take three weeks longer to reach 2 kg than a baby fed a special low birth weight formula.[18]

The initial explanation for this slower growth, proposed originally by Gordon et al[7] and by Powers[8] in America in the 1930s, and resurrected in the 1970s by Davies[3] and Fomon et al,[19] was that human milk did not contain enough protein. Decreased mineral bone content might also have contributed because accretion rates for calcium and phosphorus corresponded to only 20% and 30%, respectively, of those in utero. Critical though protein and mineral insufficiencies were in causing poor growth, this was not the only explanation. What had been overlooked in earlier studies, and came to assume greater importance, was the variable and often remarkably low fat (energy) content of donor human milk.[2] This was a major growth limiting influence.

Concern was not, however, only over short-term growth failure. Pre-term babies fed breast milk were not at increased risk of illness nor did they need to remain longer in hospital before being discharged home.[20] It was beyond dispute that their skeleton was less than optimally mineralised, but it remained to be determined whether this was harmful or permanent. The main concern was the long-term implications to future intelligence and cognitive function. In the 1970s, Dobbing and Sands in Manchester had shown that the period of maximum brain growth, the brain growth spurt, when (from extrapolation from animals) the brain was most vulnerable to damage, occurred in the latter half of gestation[21]— the development stage when pre-term babies were found not to be growing well. It had also emerged from the many classic studies of McCance and Widdowson in the 1960s and 1970s that the young of any animal species were especially vulncrable to early nutritional deficiencies.[22]

Unfortunately there was too much uncritical extrapolation from studies in small experimental animals in which definite permanent and irrecoverable damage in the long term was shown to follow less-than-adequate early nutrition. The time scale was often out of all proportion and did not take into sufficient account the differing developmental stages when inadequate nutrition had been imposed. Also, was it conceivable that a few weeks of less-than-adequate nutrition during a brain growth spurt lasting at least four years could be to the detriment both of physical growth and of neuropsychological development, as had been implied?[23] These criticisms notwithstanding, the long-term implications for psycho-motor development had become a matter of concern to clinicians, and there was seen to be an urgent need to prevent poor growth (a marker of nutritional insufficiency) and to normalise brain composition during growth.

Immunological concerns

Many paediatricians were prepared to put up with these nutritional inadequacies that led to insufficient early growth because of the umbrella of protection that was believed to be conferred by immune substances in milk—but once again research was to put a damper on the issue.

Human milk was known to contain many antimicrobial substances with the potential to prevent or modify gastrointestinal infections and possibly also respiratory tract infections. Of particular importance were milk cells, secretory IgA, lysozyme and lactoferrin. Some opinion also held that feeding breast milk lessened the risk of necrotising enterocolitis, although in the 1970s clinical evidence supporting this contention was far from conclusive.

The problem, however, was that donor milk needed to be heated before being given to the baby. Milk suckled naturally from the breast was found to contain large numbers of bacteria,[24] the predominant organisms being normal skin flora (*Staphylococcus epidermidis, Streptococcus viridans*) and some potential pathogens. Ingesting milk containing these micro-organisms was no real hazard to the healthy term baby, presumably because of specific prenatally acquired antibody protection from the mother aided by the many immune substances in breast milk. For the pre-term baby, however, deprived of much transplacental antibody and with an immune system less able to cope with potentially hostile micro-organisms, contamination of donor milk was widely presumed to be a risk factor for neonatal infection. Even with careful collection procedures which gave meticulous attention to washing and sterilising equipment, it was inevitable that micro-organisms would enter the milk. It was the presence of these micro-organisms that underlay the widespread practice of heating donor milk (other than that provided by the baby's own mother which was usually given 'raw') before feeding to babies in order to make it microbiologically 'safe'.

It was disappointing, therefore, to discover that even careful pasteurisation of human milk destroyed many of its humoral substances with powerful antimicrobial properties, with the amount of destruction directly related to the temperature to which the milk was subjected (Table 2).[25] It also appeared unlikely that any method of collecting human milk would allow the baby to receive immunologically functional cells since these were easily damaged by any

Table 2. Percentage survival of some protective antimicrobial factors in human milk after heat treatment at different temperatures (°C) for different periods of time (modified from Evans *et al*[25])

Antimicrobial factor	56° 30 min	62.5° 30 min	70° 15 min	73° 30 min	100° 3 min	100° 15 min
Immunoglobulin A	96	67–100	48	0	0	0
Lysozyme		64–100	65	2	0	3
Lactoferrin		40–100	5	1		0
Vitamin B_{12} binding capacity		52	33			43
Folic acid binding capacity		90	65			7

heat and they also adhered to the walls of the collecting and feeding bottles.

The question therefore was whether the immunological and nutritional benefits of feeding unheated donor milk outweighed the potential hazards of exposing babies to risks of illness from milk likely to be contaminated with bacteria. In less developed countries, where risks of perinatal nosocomial infection are high and with formula feeding a major risk factor for enteric disease, the strongest possible case existed to give unheated donor milk (which in most instances would be mother's own milk), providing care could be taken to express milk under the best possible hygienic conditions. In fact, the advantages conferred by feeding milk containing virtually unaltered immunological substances far outweighed the potential disadvantages of causing infection. An important study in New Delhi in 1984 by Narayanan and colleagues convincingly showed that feeding unheated expressed donor breast milk to low birth weight infants especially at risk of infection significantly diminished the incidence of systemic neonatal sepsis.[26] In more developed parts of the world, with higher standards of perinatal care and a low incidence of infection in newborn nurseries, and where formula feeding was associated with minimal risk, the anti-infective advantages of feeding raw milk were more difficult to ascertain. Some paediatricians recommended feeding babies donor human milk which had not been heated without, it was claimed, apparent ill effect. Reports of occasional outbreaks of infection on neonatal units traced to contaminated donor breast milk were made but, as a general statement, surprisingly little evidence existed linking infection in babies to feeding unheated milk.

Further doubts

By the early 1980s feeding pre-term babies donor milk had become increasingly devalued. Even feeding milk from the baby's mother was not always encouraged. Too little protein, minerals and calories and dubious antimicrobial activities combined to make this milk less than desirable. This was not sufficient, however, to discourage the publication in 1981 of a report by the Department of Health and Social Security offering practical guidelines for the collection and storage of milk for babies born pre-term and for those recovering from neonatal surgery or at risk of atopic disease.[27] But another cloud was now gathering on the horizon and fast gaining momentum—notably the concern of transmitting HIV and hepatitis B infection through breast milk. Implications for providing milk to milk banks were considerable: the complexity and expense of screening all donors for these viruses were considered hardly worth the effort, although pasteurisation of breast milk was shown to inactivate any HIV virus in the milk[28] and guidelines were made available to help in this matter.[29] At the same time, commercially available milk formulas were becoming nutritionally more sophisticated for low birth weight infants, making up for many of the nutritional defects of human milk.

A revival

Against many odds, the sacred cow that had been near to extinction was to be revived in the early 1990s, largely due to results of the multicentre study coordinated by Lucas and his colleagues in East Anglia and at the Dunn Nutrition Unit in Cambridge.[18] Having contributed to the debate in the early 1980s that described the nutritional inadequacies of human milk, these workers were now finding that it had advantages after all. In 1990 they showed that risks of necrotising enterocolitis were 6–10 times higher in pre-term babies fed formula than in those fed breast milk, including pasteurised milk.[30] Human milk was better tolerated in the first few weeks of life, pointing to a smoother gastrointestinal adaptation to enteral nutrition. A paper in 1992 by Lucas *et al.* showed cognitive function in 7–8 year old children who had received mother's milk to be better than in those who had not, possibly because of its unique blend of polyunsaturated fatty acids for optimum composition of brain cortical phospholipids.[31] Further support came from a publication from the Sorrento Hospital, Birmingham, which had continued throughout the years of uncertainty with its milk banking practices that showed milk banks still to be viable.[32] Leading articles in the *British Medical Journal*[33,34] also cautioned about the irreversible decline in the use of breast milk for pre-term babies.

Conclusion

A return to the halcyon days of milk banking is unlikely, although some large milk banks will probably maintain their activities. However, neonatal units will continue to organise their own milk kitchens with the collection and preparation of breast milk an important part of this activity. For the smallest babies it is unlikely that milk alone will be given—enrichment with supplements of protein, energy and minerals will probably be widely used. We seem therefore to have completed almost a full cycle, returning to the situation where providing a safe source of human milk, whether from the mother or from another donor, is still an essential part of health care practices for at-risk babies.

The last words on this subject have to belong to Dr Frank Ford, a paediatrician from Glasgow, who wrote the following in 1949:

> When breast milk can be obtained from a milk bank it is expensive in money and when the bank is part of the hospital's activity it is expensive in nurses' time. It is therefore essential to find out if breast milk is really so advantageous as to justify the financial outlay and the use of valuable nursing hours in collecting and processing it.[35]

I wonder if we have now reached the time when we can at last answer Ford's question and put this matter finally to rest.

References

1. Watkins AG. A breast milk bank. *The Medical Press.* March 24, 1954: 266–9
2. Gibbs JH, Fisher C, Bhattacharya S, Goddard P, Baum JD. Drip breast milk: its composition, collection and pasteurization. *Early Human Development* 1978; 227–45
3. Davies DP. Adequacy of expressed breast milk for early growth of preterm infants. *Archives of Disease in Childhood* 1977; **52**: 296–301
4. Baum JD. The effects of pasteurisation on immune factors in human milk. In: Visser HK, ed. *Nutrition and metabolism of the fetus and infant.* Boston, MA: Nijhoff, 1979: 173–83
5. Barrie H. Milk banks: in the light of history [editorial]. *Midwife, Health Visitor & Community Nurse* 1988; **24**: 243
6. Finkelstein H. *Lehrbuch der Sauglingskrankheiten.* Berlin: Springer, 1912. (Referred to by Powers, Ref. 8)
7. Gordon HH, Levine SZ, McNamara H. Feeding of premature infants: a comparison of human and cow's milk. *American Journal of Diseases of Children* 1947; **73**: 442–52
8. Powers GF. Some observations on the feeding of premature infants based on 20 years' experience at the New Haven Hospital. *Pediatrics* 1947; **1**: 145–58
9. Carroll L, Conlan D, Davies DP. Fat content of bank human milk. *Archives of Disease in Childhood* 1980; **55**: 969
10. Stocks RJP, Davies DP, Carroll L, Broderick B, Parker M. A simple method to improve the energy value of bank human milk. *Early Human Development* 1983; **8**: 175–8
11. Atkinson SA, Anderson GH, Bryan MH. Human milk: comparison of the nitrogen composition in milk from mothers of premature and full-term infants. *American Journal of Clinical Nutrition* 1980; **33**: 811–5
12. Lucas A, Suzuki S, Coombs RRA. IgA and preterm milk. *Lancet* 1982; **i**: 1242–3
13. Hamosh M, Bitman CS, Fink LM, Freed CM, *et al.* Lipid composition of preterm human milk and its digestion by the infant. In: Schaub J, ed. *Composition and physiological properties of human milk.* Amsterdam, New

York, Oxford: Elsevier Science Publishers Biomedical Division, 1985: 153–62

14. Atkinson SA, Radde IC, Chance GW, Bryan MH, Anderson GH. Macro mineral content of milk obtained during early lactation from mothers of premature infants. *Early Human Development* 1980; **4**: 5–14

15. Williamson S, Finucane E, Ellis H, Gamsu HR, *et al.* Effect of heat treatment of human milk on absorption of nitrogen, fat, sodium, calcium, and phosphorus by preterm infants. *Archives of Disease in Childhood* 1978; **53**: 555–63

16. Stocks RJ, Davies DP, Allen F, Sewell D. Loss of breast milk nutrients during tube feeding. *Archives of Disease in Childhood* 1985; **60**: 164–6

17. Brook OG, Barley J. Loss of energy during continuous infusions of breast milk. *Archives of Disease in Childhood* 1978; **53**: 344–5

18. Lucas A, Gore SM, Cole TJ, Bamford MF, *et al.* Multicentre trial on feeding low birthweight infants: effects of diet on early growth. *Archives of Disease in Childhood* 1984; **59**: 722–30

19. Fomon SJ, Ziegler EE, Vazquez HD. Human milk and the small premature infant. *American Journal of Diseases of Children* 1977; **131**: 463–7

20. Derbyshire F, Davies DP, Bacco A. Discharge of pre-term babies from neonatal units. *British Medical Journal* 1982; **284**: 233–4.

21. Dobbing J, Sands J. Quantitative growth and development of human brain. *Archives of Disease in Childhood* 1973; **48**: 757.

22. Ashwell M, ed. *McCance and Widdowson: a scientific partnership of 60 years.* London: British Nutrition Foundation, 1991

23. Tyson J, Lasky R, Mize C, White R. Growth and development of infants less than 1500 g fed bank human milk or premature formulae. *Pediatric Research* 1981; **15**: 549

24. Carroll L, Davies DP, Osman M, McNeish AS. Bacteriological criteria for feeding raw breast-milk to babies on neonatal units. *Lancet* 1979; **ii**: 732–3

25. Evans TJ, Ryley HC, Neale LM, Dodge JA, *et al.* Effect of storage and heat on antimicrobial proteins in human milk. *Archives of Disease in Childhood* 1978; **53**: 239–41

26. Narayanan I, Prakash K, Murthy NS, Gujral VV. Randomised controlled trial of effect of raw and holder pasteurised human milk and of formula supplements on incidence of neonatal infection. *Lancet* 1984; **ii**: 1111–3

27. Department of Health and Social Security. *The collection and storage of human milk.* Reports on health and social matters. London: HMSO, 1981

28. Eglin RP, Wilkinson AR. HIV infection and pasteurisation of breast milk [letter]. *Lancet* 1987; **i**: 1093

29. Department of Health and Social Security. *HIV infection, breast feeding and human milk banking.* London: HMSO, 1988 (PL/CMO (88) 13 and PH/CMO (88) 7, 27 April 1988)

30. Lucas A, Cole TJ. Breast milk and neonatal necrotising enterocolitis. *Lancet* 1990; **336**: 1519–23

31. Lucas A, Morley RTJ, Lister G, Leeson-Payne C. Breast milk and intelligence quotient in children born pre-term. *Lancet* 1992; **339**: 261–4

32. Balmer SE, Wharton BA. Human milk banking at Sorrento Maternity Hospital, Birmingham. *Archives of Disease in Childhood* 1992; **67**: 556–9

33. Williams AF. Human milk and the preterm baby: mothers should breast feed. *British Medical Journal* 1993; **306**: 1628–9
34. Davies DP. Future of human milk banks. *British Medical Journal* 1992; **305**: 433–4
35. Ford FJ. Feeding of premature babies. *Lancet* 1949; **i**: 987–94

6 | The influence of early diet on outcome in pre-term infants*

Ruth Morley
Senior Clinical Scientist, Medical Research Council Dunn Nutrition Unit &
Associate Specialist, Department of Paediatrics, Addenbrooke's Hospital, Cambridge

Alan Lucas
*Head of Infant and Child Nutrition Group, Medical Research Council Dunn
Nutrition Unit, Cambridge*

There has been considerable interest in the concept of programming, defined by Lucas as the process whereby a stimulus or insult applied at a critical or sensitive period of development results in a long-term or permanent effect on the structure or function of the organism.[1] There is substantial evidence from animal studies that programming does occur and can profoundly affect structure or function in adult life.[1,2] More recently, epidemiological studies have suggested that nutritional influences operating during intra-uterine and early postnatal life could have long-term consequences for blood pressure, diabetes and ischaemic heart disease.[3]

It is of concern to neonatologists that suboptimal nutrition during early life could have long-term consequences for neurodevelopment in infants born pre-term. There is evidence that animals fed low nutrient diets at a critical period of early brain development have reduced brain size and brain cell number. However, Smart, in a review of 165 reported animal studies,[4] did not find a consistent disadvantage in later performance for undernourished animals when compared with well-nourished controls.

A number of studies of malnourished children, mainly from third world countries, have drawn differing conclusions regarding the relationship between early diet and later developmental status.[5] Some show a developmental benefit for children receiving dietary supplements, while others have shown similar benefits from dietary supplements combined with infant stimulation programmes or from infant stimulation alone. Most of these studies have been retrospective and confounded by social and environmental depriva-

*Reproduced by permission of *Acta Paediatrica*.

tion, the effects of which may also be modified by interventions.

Pre-term children are a uniquely suitable group in which to test the concept of developmental programming by early nutrition because they are born at a stage of rapid brain growth and maturation. More importantly, when these studies were planned in the early 1980s there was no general agreement on the optimal feeding regimen for pre-term infants. In practice, enteral diets used differed widely in nutrient content, ranging from unsupplemented donor milk to nutrient-enriched formula designed to meet the calculated nutritional needs of pre-term infants. With such a lack of agreement, it was not only practical and ethical to conduct randomised studies of the effect of early nutrition on later developmental status but also important as a guide to clinical management.

We conducted trials of pre-term infant feeding in five centres in the UK, enrolling 926 infants with birth weights under 1,850 g, with randomisation as shown in Figure 1. Study 1 was conducted in three centres with donor breast milk banks (Cambridge, Ipswich and King's Lynn), and study 2 in Norwich and Sheffield, centres without breast milk banks. In each study mothers were asked whether they wished to provide their own expressed breast milk for their infants. If they elected to do this, their infant was randomly allocated the trial diet as a supplement, to ensure adequate enteral intake when the expressed breast milk was not sufficient. If the mother did not wish to express her milk, the infant was allocated the trial diet as the sole milk source.

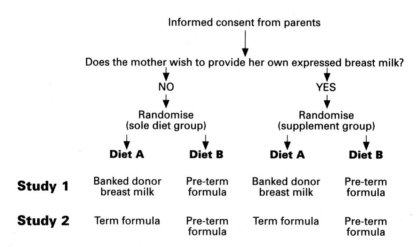

Randomisation was stratified by birth weight. Infants under 1,200 g were randomised separately.

Fig. 1. *Study design.*

Table 1. Major nutrient contents of diets of pre-term infants

Per 100 ml	Pre-term formula	Term formula	Mother's expressed breast milk*	Banked donor breast milk*
Protein (g)	2.0	1.5	1.5	1.1
Fat (g)	4.9	3.8	3.0	1.7
Carbohydrate (g)	7.0	7.0	7.0	7.1
kcal	80	68	62	46
Sodium (mg)	45	19	23	16
Calcium (mg)	70	35	35	35
Phosphorus (mg)	35	29	15	15

*Mean values from analysis of pooled samples.

In study 1 the dietary comparison was between A, banked donor breast milk, and B, a pre-term formula designed to meet the nutritional needs of pre-term infants (Osterprem, Crookes Healthcare Ltd). There were 159 subjects randomised in the sole diet group and 343 whose randomised diet was as a supplement to mother's milk. In study 2 the comparison was between A, standard term formula (Osterfeed, now Ostermilk, Crookes Healthcare Ltd), and B, the pre-term formula as above, with 160 subjects in the sole diet group and 264 in the supplement group. The major nutrient contents of these diets are shown in Table 1.

Infants were fed the assigned diet until they reached 2,000 g in weight or were discharged from the neonatal unit, whichever was first. After leaving the study there was no further influence on the infants' diet; they were fed as their parents chose.

Outcome in the neonatal period

Mortality and morbidity

There were no differences between any of the randomised comparisons in terms of mortality or respiratory morbidity. However, there was a higher incidence of confirmed necrotising enterocolitis in those fed pre-term formula (4/76) as sole diet than in those fed banked donor milk (1/86) as sole diet. In the non-random

Table 2. Diet and confirmed necrotising enterocolitis (NEC)

Diet	No. of infants	NEC (%)
Term formula or pre-term formula as sole diets	236	7.2
Term or pre-term formula as supplements to mother's expressed breast milk	437	2.5
Banked pasteurised donor breast milk as sole diet	86	1.2
Banked pasteurised donor breast milk as supplement to mother's expressed breast milk	170	1.2

comparison shown in Table 2 there is a clear benefit from human milk. Those fed only human milk, either as banked donor milk alone or as a supplement to mother's expressed milk, had the lowest incidence of confirmed necrotising enterocolitis, whereas those fed only formula had the highest incidence.[6]

Growth

There were considerable differences between the diet groups. In study 1, overall, those fed pre-term formula had significantly higher steady-state weight and length gains than those fed donor milk.[7] The greatest differences were seen in the comparison between pre-term formula and donor milk as sole diets—pre-term formula fed infants regained their birth weight in a median of 10 days compared with 16 days for those fed donor milk. Infants fed the pre-term formula also had faster gains in head circumference and in calculated brain weight than those fed donor milk.

In study 2, differences between diet groups were less marked, but those fed pre-term formula had faster steady-state weight gain than those fed term formula. When these formulas were compared as sole diets, the pre-term formula fed children had faster head circumference gain.[8]

Using data from study 1 it has been calculated that, for example, a typical infant born at 28 weeks of gestation (weighing 1,000 g) would take 47 days to reach 2,000 g on pre-term formula compared with 68 days on donor breast milk.[7] Infants fed a nutrient enriched pre-term formula are therefore likely to be discharged home sooner, with benefits not only for the child and his family but also for health care resources.

Long-term outcome measures

Developmental outcome at nine months post-term

All outcome measures in these studies were undertaken by assessors blind to the dietary allocation.

Children from study 1 were assessed at nine months post-term using the Knobloch, Pasamanick and Sherard developmental screening inventory. Those fed pre-term formula had significant advantages in the adaptive, language and personal/social areas of development compared with those fed donor milk.[9] There was a significant advantage for pre-term formula fed infants in overall developmental quotient (DQ) (mean DQ, 100.4 (SE 0.78) compared with 97.9 (SE 0.74) in those fed donor milk).

The developmental advantage of pre-term formula was greater in some subgroups. There was a significant interaction between the dietary effect on development and size for gestation, with a significantly greater benefit from pre-term formula for a child born small for gestation (eg a 5.3 point advantage in children born less than the 10th centile). The advantage was also greater in males than in females, though the interaction was not statistically significant.

Developmental outcome at 18 months post-term

Children from both studies were examined at 18 months post-term and assessed using the Bayley scales of infant development. This test has mental and motor scales, from which are derived the mental development index (MDI) and the psychomotor development index (PDI). Study 2 was completed first[8] and showed a significant advantage in PDI for children fed pre-term rather than term formula, with the greatest advantage when these diets were compared as sole diets. Subgroup analyses again showed that the advantage was greater in male than in female children and in those born small rather than with appropriate weights for gestation. In this study, therefore, there were significant interactions both between diet and sex and between diet and size for gestation, showing that the advantage from pre-term formula was significantly greater in males than in females and in children born small, rather than the appropriate weight for gestation.

Many infants received little of the assigned diet, in some cases because their mothers were able to express enough breast milk to satisfy most of the infant's needs, and in others because the infant was very sick and was fed parenterally for a prolonged period. In the children who had received over 50% of their intake as trial diet and who had received at least two weeks of full enteral feeds during the trial, a significant advantage for children fed pre-term formula was seen in both motor and mental development; those fed pre-term formula had a mean MDI score of 103.9 (SE 1.9) and a PDI score of 97.7 (SE 2.1) compared with MDI 96.3 (SE 1.9) and PDI 88.2 (SE 1.8) in those fed the standard term formula (p <0.05 and p <0.001, respectively). In contrast to these findings from study 2, there were only small developmental differences at 18 months between the diet groups in study 1.[10] This was surprising because the banked donor milk had the lowest nutrient content (lower than the term formula).

Human milk and development

The possibility was considered that human milk may contain factors which are important for brain growth and maturation, thus accounting for the relatively small differences in study 1 compared with the larger differences seen when term and pre-term formula were compared as sole diets (in study 2).[10] In this latter comparison, neither group received any human milk and the difference between the allocated diets was in nutrient content.

Mothers were asked prior to randomisation whether or not they wished to provide their milk for their infants. Developmental scores at 18 months were significantly higher in children whose mothers chose to provide their milk.[11] Children from both studies have now been assessed using a short form of the revised anglicised version of the Weschler intelligence scale for children at 7.5–8 years of age. Interim analysis again showed a significant advantage in intelligence quotient for those whose mothers expressed milk.[12] Even after adjusting for the considerable social and demographic differences that we have shown exist between mothers who choose to provide their milk compared to those who do not,[13] significant advantages remain for those infants whose mothers choose to express milk.

There are several possible explanations for these findings:

- that we failed to identify all relevant social differences between the populations and therefore failed to 'adjust out' the advantage;
- that the mother's choice to express her milk reflected her level of concern for the infant's welfare, later reflected in her stimulation of the child's development; or
- that there are factors in human milk which promote brain growth or development.

In support of the latter, we found that in the groups whose mothers chose *not* to provide their milk (sole diet comparisons form studies 1 and 2) there was a developmental advantage for children fed donor milk compared with those fed term formula, despite the lower nutrient content of the former.

Human milk contains long-chain fatty acids, notably docosahexaenoic and arachidonic acids which are found in abundance in the brain and the retina. These were not present in significant amounts in the cow's milk formulas. There are also many biologically active peptides in human milk whose roles are little understood.

There is conflicting evidence from population studies, but some have found a developmental advantage in breast-fed children born at term, even after adjusting for social and demographic differences between the families of those fed breast milk versus formula. It is likely, however, that any candidate nutrient or non-nutrient factors in human milk would be of more importance in the pre-term infant born at a time of rapid brain growth and maturation.

Human milk and bone mineral content

A subgroup of children from study 1 living near the hospital in Cambridge were seen between 4.5 and 5.9 years of age for assessment of their bone mineral content. This work was undertaken by Dr N Bishop who, interestingly, found that the proportion of mother's milk in the infant's diet influences bone mineral content positively many years later, irrespective of body size.[14] Although the differences in calcium and phosphate content between donor milk and pre-term formula may be important, it is also possible that there is a non-nutrient factor in human milk that influences later bone mineralisation. Further studies will be conducted to determine whether this effect persists into adult life.

Conclusions

Despite intensive research in infant nutrition over the past 50 years, uncertainty exists in nearly every major area of practice. A key factor in this uncertainty has been the lack of knowledge on whether diet or nutritional status in early life has a long-term or permanent influence on health, growth or performance. The possibility that early nutrition has long-term consequences in man has been much debated. There have been limited opportunities to perform formal randomised studies on the effect of early nutrition in man, and many studies have been flawed by problems with study design. Infants born pre-term are a special group. At the start of our study in 1982 evidence on which to base choice of diet was inconsistent and related only to short-term outcome, and diets available for such babies differed greatly in nutrient content. It was both ethical and practical to conduct a formal, randomised trial of early diet and outcome in this group and the results were clearly needed for management decisions.

We have undertaken a long-term prospective outcome study on 926 pre-term infants randomly assigned to the diet received in the neonatal period. Surviving children have been followed at nine and 18 months and now at 7.5–8 years of age. From our studies up to 18 months post-term we have found evidence that early diet has long-term effects on developmental status. Children born small for gestation and male children were especially vulnerable to the effects of poor early diet. Preliminary analyses of data from the 7.5–8 year assessment of these children suggest that some of the dietary effects on development are persisting well into childhood. Our findings suggest that human milk may contain factors which promote brain growth or development and also bone mineralisation later in childhood. If confirmed, these data will provide evidence that a brief period of dietary manipulation, on average during only the first four weeks of life, influences development many years later.

Our studies would support the view that human milk is beneficial for the health and development of children born pre-term. Furthermore, those fed a nutrient enriched pre-term formula have performed better generally than those fed a standard term formula, either as sole diet or supplement to mother's milk.

We plan long-term follow-up of this cohort to investigate the influence of early diet on performance and health in adult life.

References

1. Lucas A. Programming by early nutrition in man. In: Bock GR, Whelan J, eds. *The childhood environment and adult disease* (CIBA Foundation Symposium 156). Chichester: Wiley, 1991: 38–55
2. Lewis DS, Mott GE, McMahan CA Masoro EJ, *et al.* Deferred effects of preweaning diet on atherosclerosis in adolescent baboons. *Arteriosclerosis* 1988; **8**: 274–80
3. Barker DJP, Gluckman PD, Godfrey KM, Harding JE, *et al.* Fetal nutrition and cardiovascular disease in adult life. *Lancet* 1993; **341**: 938–41
4. Smart J. Undernutrition, learning and memory: review of experimental studies. In: Taylor TG, Jenkins NK, eds. *Proceedings of XIII International Congress of Nutrition.* London: John Libbey, 1986: 74–8

5. Grantham McGregor S. *Field studies in early nutrition and later achievement.* London: Academic Press, 1987: 221–33

6. Lucas A, Cole TJ. Breast milk and necrotising enterocolitis. *Lancet* 1990; **336**: 1519–23

7. Lucas A, Gore SM. Multicentre trial on feeding low birthweight infants: effects of diet on early growth. *Archives of Disease in Childhood* 1984; **59**: 722–30

8. Lucas A, Morley R, Cole TJ, Gore SM, *et al.* Early diet in preterm babies and developmental status at 18 months. *Lancet* 1990; **335**: 1477–81

9. Lucas A, Morley R, Cole TJ, Gore SM, *et al.* Early diet in preterm babies and developmental status in infancy. *Archives of Disease in Childhood* 1989; **64**: 1570–8

10. Lucas A, Morley R, Cole TJ, Gore SM. A randomised multicentre study of human milk versus formula and later development in preterm infants. *Archives of Disease in Childhood* 1994; **70**: F141–6

11. Morley R, Cole TJ, Powell R, Lucas A. Mother's choice to provide breast milk and developmental outcome. *Archives of Disease in Childhood* 1988; **63**: 1382–5

12. Lucas A, Morley R, Cole TJ, Lister G, Leeson-Payne C. Breast milk and subsequent intelligence quotient in children born preterm. *Lancet* 1992; **339**: 261–4

13. Lucas A, Cole TJ, Morley R, Lucas PJ, *et al.* Factors associated with material choice to provide breast milk for low birthweight infants. *Archives of Disease in Childhood* 1988; **63**: 48–52

14. Bishop N. *Bone mineralisation in infants born preterm: effect of early diet.* MD Thesis, Victoria University of Manchester, 1993

7 | Early nutrition and coronary heart disease

David J P Barker
Professor of Clinical Epidemiology, University of Southampton; Director, Medical Research Council Environmental Epidemiology Unit, Southampton General Hospital

Recent research has shown that babies who are small at birth and during infancy will be at increased risk of developing coronary heart disease, stroke, diabetes or hypertension during adult life. That a person's destiny and lifespan may be determined before birth is well known. Genetically determined diseases such as Huntington's chorea illustrate how a long period of normal development and adult life can be prematurely brought to an end by the action of inherited defects. What is new is the realisation that it is not only the presence or absence of genes that controls our destiny but the way in which gene expression may be permanently changed by the nutrient environment in early life.

There are three reasons why this new field of research has developed:

1. The current explanation of coronary heart disease, a 'destructive' model in which inappropriate adult lifestyles hasten ageing processes, fails to account for either the time trends of the disease or its geography, or why one person gets the disease and another does not.
2. The search for alternative explanations led to a strong geographical clue that the role of fetal life in the genesis of coronary heart disease might be much greater than had been thought.[1]
3. Animal experiments show that changes in nutrition in early life permanently change the growth and form of the body together with a range of its structures and functions.[2] This phenomenon is known as 'programming'.

Studies in animals

The substantial body of evidence on the plasticity of the fetus, its ability to adapt to undernutrition, and the permanent effects of these adaptations, derives from animal experiments carried out by Widdowson and others.[2] These studies allow us to make two predictions about the human fetus:

1. Lack of nutrients or oxygen will cause persisting changes, which include altered metabolism, including glucose and lipid metabolism, altered blood pressure and 'settings' of hormonal axes, enzymes and cell receptors.

2. The long-term effects of undernutrition depend on the stage at which it occurs. Tissues and systems tend to be vulnerable to programming during phases of rapid cell replication, and different tissues undergo these 'sensitive' phases of development at different times.

Small size at birth and in infancy

It has been possible to explore the links between growth *in utero* and later coronary heart disease as a result of a search of the archives in Britain which revealed collections of birth records of men and women born 50 years and more ago in Hertfordshire, Preston and Sheffield. Figure 1 shows findings in a group of 8,175 men born in the county of Hertfordshire before 1930. Their weight at one year of age strongly predicted their subsequent death rates from coronary heart disease.[3] Death rates fell steeply between those who were small and those who were large at one year. There were similar trends in coronary heart disease with birth weight in men and women. A study in Sheffield showed that the small babies with high coronary death rates in adulthood were small in relation to duration of gestation rather than because they were prematurely born.

These findings pose the question of what are the processes linking reduced early growth with adult disease. Examination of samples from men and women who were born and still live in Hertfordshire, Sheffield and Preston shows that babies who were small have, as adults, raised blood pressure, raised serum cholesterol and plasma fibrinogen concentrations, and impaired glucose tolerance[4]—the main risk factors for coronary heart disease. Table 1 shows the mean systolic pressures of men and women aged 64–71 years. Systolic pressure falls progressively between those who were small at birth and those who were large. This relationship between birth weight and blood pressure has now been demonstrated in 19 studies of children and adults, and there is a secure base for saying that impaired fetal growth is strongly linked to blood pressure at all ages except during adolescence, when the tracking of blood

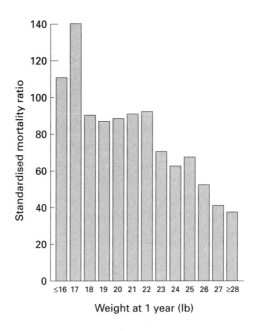

Fig. 1.   *Standardised mortality ratios for coronary heart disease in 8,175 men born during 1911–30 according to their weight at one year of age.*

Table 1. Mean systolic pressure (mmHg) in men and women aged 64–71 years according to birth weight

Birth weight			
(lb)	(kg)	Men	Women
≤5.5	≤2.50	171 (18)	169 (9)
→6.5	→2.95	168 (53)	165 (33)
→7.5	→3.41	168 (144)	160 (68)
→8.5	→3.86	165 (111)	163 (48)
>8.5	>3.86	163 (92)	155 (26)
Total		*166 (418)*	*161 (184)*
Standard deviation		24	26

Figures in brackets are numbers of subjects.

pressure levels which begins in early childhood is perturbed by the adolescent growth spurt. Differences in blood pressure associated with birth weight are small in childhood but are magnified throughout life, suggesting that there may be amplification as well as initiation processes. It is not known what initiates high blood pressure in intra-uterine life, but there are interesting clues, including the work of Edwards, Seckl and colleagues in Edinburgh which has pointed to the possible role of cortisol.[5]

Table 2 shows the prevalence of non-insulin dependent diabetes and impaired glucose tolerance according to birth weight in a group of men in Hertfordshire.[6] The prevalence falls sharply between men who were small at birth and those who were large. There are similar findings in women. This association between birth weight and diabetes has been replicated in two other studies in Britain, two studies in the USA, and one in Sweden.

Body proportions at birth

Studies of men and women who were small at birth have shown that they are resistant to insulin. The occurrence of insulin resistance in adults is characterised in a syndrome, syndrome X, in which diabetes, hypertension and raised plasma triglyceride concentrations coincide. Allowing for current body mass, the relative risk of having syndrome X among people 6.5 lb (2.95 kg) or less at birth is about

Table 2. Prevalence of non-insulin dependent diabetes and impaired glucose tolerance in men aged 59–70 years according to birth weight

Birth weight (lb)*	Number of men	% with impaired glucose tolerance or diabetes	Odds ratio adjusted for body mass index (95% confidence interval)
≤5.5	20	40	6.6(1.5–28)
→6.5	47	34	4.8(1.3–17)
→7.5	104	31	4.6(1.4–16)
→8.5	117	22	2.6(0.8–8.9)
→9.5 (4.31 kg)	54	13	1.4(0.3–5.6)
>9.5	28	14	1.0
Total	*370*	*25*	

*See Table 1 for birth weights in kilograms.

10 times higher than among people who were more than 9.5 lb (4.31 kg) Table 3. This is a large difference in risk. For comparison, the risk of coronary heart disease among smokers compared with non-smokers is about 2. The insulin resistance syndrome is associated not only with low birthweight but also with thinness at birth, as measured by a low ponderal index (birth weight/length^3). Babies who are thin at birth lack muscle as well as fat, and muscle in adult life is the peripheral site of insulin action. Insulin tolerance tests on men and women aged 50 confirm that those who were thin at birth are less sensitive to insulin.

Raised blood pressure in adult life is associated with both thinness at birth and short body length in relation to head size. Short babies are thought to have encountered undernutrition in late gestation and to have sustained brain growth at the expense of the trunk, including the abdominal viscera. An analysis of mean serum cholesterol concentrations in a group of men and women aged about 50 showed that total and low density lipoprotein (LDL) cholesterol concentrations fall between people who had small and large abdominal circumferences at birth (Table 4).[7] Abdominal circumference reflects liver size, the liver being disproportionately large in the fetus. An inference from Table 4 is that babies with impaired liver development permanently reset their cholesterol metabolism. Reduced abdominal circumference at birth is also associated with raised plasma concentrations of fibrinogen, another

Table 3. Prevalence of syndrome X (type 2 diabetes, hypertension and hyperlipidaemia) in men according to birth weight

Birth weight (lb)*	Total number of men	% with syndrome X	Odds ratio adjusted for body mass index (95% confidence interval)
≤5.5	20	30	18.0(2.6–118)
→6.5	54	19	8.4(1.5–49)
→7.5	114	17	8.5(1.5–46)
→8.5	123	12	4.9(0.9–27)
→9.5	64	6	2.2(0.3–14)
>9.5	32	6	1.0
Total	*407*	*14*	

*See Tables 1 and 2 for birth weights in kilograms.

Table 4. Mean serum lipid concentrations according to abdominal circumference at birth in men and women aged 50–53 years

Abdominal circumference (in)	(cm)	Number of people	Total cholesterol (mmol/l)	LDL cholesterol (mmol/l)
≤11.5	29.21	53	6.7	4.5
→12.0	30.48	43	6.9	4.6
→12.5	31.75	31	6.8	4.4
→13.0	33.02	45	6.2	4.0
>13.0	33.02	45	6.1	4.0
Total		*217*	*6.5*	*4.3*

strong predictor of coronary heart disease. The differences in serum cholesterol and plasma fibrinogen concentrations associated with the range of abdominal circumference at birth are large, equivalent to at least a 30% difference in risk of coronary heart disease.

Other observations suggest that infant feeding may also programme adult cholesterol metabolism. Men in Hertfordshire who were breast-fed beyond one year were found to have raised serum LDL cholesterol concentrations and increased death rates from coronary heart disease.[8] The mechanisms by which late weaning of infants might programme lipid metabolism are a matter for speculation. One possible explanation, however, which derives from observations on baboons, is that thyroid hormones present in breast milk may down-regulate the suckling infant's thyroid function and thereby influence cholesterol metabolism.

Summary of programming

This brief review allows a number of conclusions.

1. Restriction of nutrients or oxygen *in utero* leaves permanent marks on the physiology and structure of the body. As an example, Table 5 shows the blood pressures of the offspring of four groups of pregnant rats given varying amounts of dietary protein.[9] The offspring of the rats given lower protein diets had raised blood pressure nine weeks after birth, and this persisted through adult life.

2. Experiments on animals have established that undernutrition at different times in early life has different effects. In early gestation, it leads to proportionate loss of body size, as in the proportionately

Table 5. Effects of fetal exposure to maternal low protein diets on systolic blood pressure in adult rats

Dietary protein (% by weight of food intake)	Number of rats	Mean (SD) systolic blood pressure 9 weeks after birth (mm Hg)
18	15	137 (± 4)
12	13	152 (± 3)
9	13	153 (± 3)
6	11	159 (± 3)

small newborn human baby. In late gestation, undernutrition leads to disproportionate growth, as in the thin or short human baby. Disproportionate growth rather than small size seems to hold a key to the origins of coronary heart disease. Twenty years ago Widdowson showed that undernutrition could effect profound changes in the relative size of the body's organs without any major change in overall body size.[2]

3. The rapidly growing baby is more vulnerable to undernutrition. When rickets was common 70 years ago it was not small babies who got the disease but larger, more rapidly growing ones. Slow growth protects against undernutrition. In some countries such as China, where proportionate intra-uterine growth retardation is widespread, coronary heart disease is rare. Growth retardation in China seems to lead to down-regulation of growth in early gestation, which could protect the fetus from the effects of undernutrition later in gestation, and from the development of the disproportion associated with coronary heart disease.

4. Fetal undernutrition, which programmes the body, itself results from inadequate maternal intake of food or from inadequate transport or transfer of nutrients. Studies of the birth weights of families show a strong correlation between the birth weights of people related through their mothers, but not between those of people related only through their fathers. This and other findings suggest that fetal growth is not predominantly controlled by the fetal genome but by the supply of nutrients and oxygen from the mother.[8] For a period of seven months in 1944 there was an embargo on food supplies to the population of western Holland, and people starved. Something is now known about what happened in adulthood to the generation of babies conceived or born during this famine.[10] Girls conceived in the famine but born after libera-

tion by the Allies had normal birth weight and grew up to be normal women, but their babies, when they were born, were small. It seems that the ability of these women to deliver nutrients to their babies had been impaired by their own fetal experience. This observation illustrates how fetal nutrition depends not only on what the mother eats during pregnancy but on her physiological and metabolic competence established during her early life, as well as her nutrient stores before pregnancy.

Another aspect of the complex links between maternal and fetal nutrition is shown in Table 6, in which the mean systolic blood pressures of a group of men and women are arranged by four groups of birth weight and four groups of placental weight.[11] As expected from previous findings, those people with a heavier birth weight had lower blood pressure but, unexpectedly, at any birth weight men and women who had had larger placentas had higher blood pressure. From studies in animals, placental enlargement is known to be an adaptation to lack of nutrients including oxygen. In humans, three kinds of baby are known to have disproportionately large placentas: the offspring of mothers who are anaemic in pregnancy, who exercise during pregnancy or who live at high altitude.[8] The fetus seems to attempt to overcome the deficiency in its supply of nutrients or oxygen by increasing the area of its attachment to the mother. A high ratio of placental weight to birth weight is linked to cardiovascular disease, impaired glucose tolerance and raised plasma fibrinogen concentrations in later life as well as to hypertension. The placenta seems to play an important role in programming the baby.

New model of coronary heart disease

A new model for the causation of coronary heart disease is emerging.[8] Under the old model, an inappropriate lifestyle, including cigarette smoking and lack of exercise, leads to accelerated destruction of the body in middle and late life, including the more rapid development of atheroma, raised blood pressure and the development of insulin resistance. Under the new model, coronary heart disease results not primarily from external forces but from the body's self organisation, that is homoeostatic settings of enzyme activity, cell receptors and hormone feedback, which are established in response to undernutrition *in utero* and lead eventually to premature death.

Table 6. Mean systolic blood pressure (mm Hg) of men and women aged 46–54 according to placental weight and birth weight

Birth weight (lb)*	Placental weight (lb)				
	≤1.0	→1.25	→1.5	>1.5	All
<5.5	152 (26)	154 (13)	153 (5)	206 (1)	154 (45)
→6.5	147 (16)	151 (54)	150 (28)	166 (8)	151 (106)
→7.5	144 (20)	148 (77)	145 (45)	160 (27)	149 (169)
>7.5	133 (6)	148 (27)	147 (42)	154 (54)	149 (129)
All	147 (68)	149 (171)	147 (120)	157 (90)	150 (449)

Figures in brackets are numbers of subjects.
*See Table 1 for birth weights in kilograms.

References

1. Barker DJP, Osmond C. Infant mortality, childhood nutrition, and ischaemic heart disease in England and Wales. *Lancet* 1986; i: 1977–81
2. McCance RA, Widdowson EM. The determinants of growth and form. *Proceedings of the Royal Society of London.* 1974; **B185**: 1–17
3. Osmond C, Barker DJP, Winter PD, Fall CHD, Simmonds SJ. Early growth and death from cardiovascular disease in women. *British Medical Journal* 1993; **307**: 1519–24
4. Barker DJP, Gluckman PD, Godfrey KM, Harding JE, *et al.* Fetal nutrition and cardiovascular disease in adult life. *Lancet* 1993; **341**: 938–41
5. Benediktsson R, Lindsay RS, Noble J, Seckl JR, Edwards CRW. Glucocorticoid exposure *in utero:* new model for adult hypertension. *Lancet* 1993; **341**: 339–41.
6. Hales CN, Barker DJP, Clark PMS, Cox LJ, *et al.* Fetal and infant growth and impaired glucose tolerance at age 64. *British Medical Journal* 1991 **303**: 1019–22
7. Barker DJP, Martyn CN, Osmond C, Hales CN, *et al.* Growth *in utero* and serum cholesterol concentrations in adult life. *British Medical Journal* 1993; **307**: 1524–7
8. Barker DJP. *Mothers, babies and disease in later life.* London: British Medical Journal Books, 1994
9. Langley SC, Jackson AA. Increased systolic blood pressure in adult rats induced by fetal exposure to maternal low protein diets. *Clinical Science* 1994; **86**: 217–22
10. Lumey LH. Decreased birthweights in infants after maternal *in utero* exposure to the Dutch famine of 1944–45. *Paediatric and Perinatal Epidemiology* 1992; **6**: 240–53
11. Barker DJP, Bull AR, Osmond C, Simmonds SJ. Fetal and placental size and risk of hypertension in adult life. *British Medical Journal* 1990; **301**: 259–62

8 | Intra-uterine growth retardation: achieving 'catch-up'

Michael Cosgrove
Lecturer, University Department of Child Health, University of Wales College of Medicine, Cardiff

> There are tiny, puny infants with great vitality. Their movements are untiring and their crying lusty, for their organs are quite capable of performing their allotted functions. These infants will live, for although their weight is inferior ... their sojourn in the womb was longer.[1]

The recognition that some babies are born small not because of premature birth but because of poor intra-uterine growth gained wide acceptance only just over 30 years ago. Over about the last 20 years the main focus of neonatal research has been firmly on infants born prematurely, with infants born at term with intra-uterine growth retardation (IUGR) attracting rather less interest. Recent years have, however, seen much epidemiological attention focused on links between early (ie fetal and infant) life and diseases of middle and late adult life. Professor David Barker has proposed the theory that factors acting in fetal and infant life may be important in programming abnormal physiology and metabolism, thereby increasing the risk of diabetes mellitus and cardiovascular and respiratory disease in adult life.[2] The implications of this for future health planning have again stimulated interest in the prevention and early management of IUGR.

This chapter describes the aetiology, recognition and importance of IUGR, the process of catch-up growth and factors which may limit it, and suggests possible nutritional strategies which may optimise catch-up growth following IUGR.

Aetiology of intra-uterine growth retardation

Infants may be born small at term because of a reduced growth potential or because of what Gruenwald describes as an insufficient supply line.[3] Examples of conditions causing the former are genetic factors, major congenital malformations, chromosomal abnormalities and early intra-uterine infection with rubella, cytomegalovirus and toxoplasma. The majority of small-for-dates infants show evidence of fetal malnutrition, often for no obvious reason. They will therefore have a low weight, out of proportion to the reduction in their length and head circumference. Clinically they are recognised as wasted infants with reduced body fat and muscle bulk (Figure 1).

Fetal malnutrition is the result of an inadequate supply line, because of either maternal problems or impaired function of the placenta. Maternal hypertension and cigarette smoking in pregnancy can both cause IUGR through their effects on placental perfusion. Maternal diseases, particularly cardiac and renal disease, are also associated with impaired fetal growth. Rate of intra-uterine growth is impaired in multiple pregnancies after 29–32 weeks gestation, probably by a process of the fetal demands outstripping the

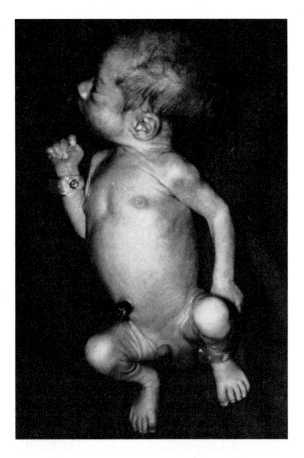

Fig. 1. *An infant born at full term showing typical features of intra-uterine malnutrition, muscle wasting and lack of subcutaneous fat.*

supply line's capacity. Severe maternal nutritional insufficiency affects fetal growth in developing countries. For example, it is estimated that in parts of India up to 40% of all infants are of low birth weight due principally to maternal undernutrition,[4] but this is rare in Western nations.

Problems associated with the placenta which may affect fetal growth include abnormal sites of insertion, and long-standing premature separation of a significant portion of the placenta leading to an infarct of the affected portion. King and Loke have recently proposed that idiopathic IUGR is due to poor development of the maternal blood supply to the fetoplacental unit because of defective interaction between placental trophoblast cells and cells of the maternal uterine mucosa (the decidua).[5]

Recognition of intra-uterine growth retardation

The antenatal detection of the infant who is small for gestational age (SGA) or, perhaps more importantly, whose growth is faltering is one of the prime objectives of modern obstetric care because of the well-known increased risk of perinatal morbidity and mortality. Ultrasound is generally regarded as the most sensitive method, with reference standards available for several geometric parameters. Serial ultrasonic measurements are better than a single measurement at diagnosing fetal growth retardation, as confirmed by neonatal morphometry.

In clinical practice, assessment of fetal growth usually ignores maternal physiological variables known to affect it (eg maternal weight and height, ethnic origin, parity). Gardosi *et al.* have constructed a computer generated antenatal chart 'customised' for each individual pregnancy which allows for these factors.[6] When these adjusted centiles were compared with conventional standards, a large proportion of babies were found to be incorrectly classified as IUGR when their growth was normal, and vice versa, on conventional charts.

At birth, IUGR is conventionally recognised on the basis of low birth weight for gestational age. However, there is variation both in the population standards used and in the centile chosen as the cut-off. In addition, low birth weight for gestational age is not interchangeable with IUGR; some infants with a genetic potential for larger than average growth may suffer intra-uterine malnutrition but still have a birth weight greater than the tenth centile. Conversely, an infant who is genetically small may have an optimal intra-uterine environment but still be below the third centile at birth.

Recognition that a low birth weight for a given gestational age *per se* is not necessarily indicative of IUGR has prompted the search for others markers. Perhaps the most useful of these is the ponderal index (weight in grams $\times 100/\text{length}^3$) which relates birth weight to length, and so is a measure of leanness. This index will be low in infants with wasting of muscle and subcutaneous tissue, usually due to late third trimester growth retardation, but normal in infants with a symmetric pattern of growth retardation, usually associated with impairment of growth from earlier in pregnancy. Other proposed markers of late gestation growth retardation include a reduced ratio of mid-arm to head circumference, reduced skinfold thickness and altered body composition, with a relative increase in extracellular fluid.

Importance of intra-uterine growth retardation

IUGR infants are more likely to suffer intrapartum asphyxia, and hypoglycaemia and polycythaemia in the neonatal period. They continue to be at increased vulnerability beyond the neonatal period, with an increased infant mortality rate and increased morbidity in the first year of life.

As a group, IUGR infants remain lighter and shorter in later childhood than a group of infants of average birth weight. However, there are large variations between individual infants, with those whose IUGR commences in the second trimester, shown by early slowing of skull growth on serial ultrasonic cephalometry, more likely to have a height and weight less than the tenth centile as young children.[7]

Increasing recognition of the importance of fetal and infant nutrition on the developing brain has led to concern over the neurodevelopmental outcome of IUGR infants. The period of intra-uterine malnutrition accounts for only a small proportion of the total period of rapid brain growth in humans, but it is the part containing the period of maximum acceleration, and thus it has greater vulnerability to any growth-inhibiting process. The work of Dobbing[8] and the theory of programming, suggesting that an early insult operating at a critical period may result in a long-term change in the structure or function of the developing organism, might be expected to predict that neurological development will be retarded following IUGR.

Several studies have shown that SGA infants have significant developmental retardation, and are particularly prone to minimal cerebral dysfunction characterised by hyperactivity, short attention span, learning difficulties, poor fine coordination and hyper-reflexia.[9] Postnatal developmental progress may be related to timing of onset of growth failure, with early onset IUGR more likely to be followed by slow development.[7]

Finally, the recent studies on the role of factors affecting the fetus in adult disease suggest that the IUGR infant remains significantly disadvantaged up to and beyond middle age, with possible increased risks of cardiovascular, respiratory and metabolic diseases.[2]

Catch-up growth

Failure of growth in infancy and childhood is a response to many different pathological states. A common response seen when the cause of the growth failure is treated or removed is that growth resumes at a rate well in excess of that which would be expected for the age or maturity of the child. This phase of recovery has been called 'catch-up' growth.[10] When applied to the postnatal growth of infants subjected to intra-uterine malnutrition, birth is the event which removes the constraint of the adverse intra-uterine environment. Catch-up growth is then an attempt to recover, in a short period after birth, the prenatal growth deficit (Figure 2).

Several studies on catch-up growth in the early postnatal period in SGA infants have found that it is not uniform. This is not surprising, given that, by aetiology, they are such a heterogeneous group. Thus, while some infants' postnatal growth reverts rapidly towards the mean, others continue with slow postnatal growth, reflecting their intra-uterine growth pattern.[11] Acceleration of growth in weight, when compared with national standards, begins soon after birth and continues for an average of six months when it returns to a rate similar to that of appropriately sized infants. Acceleration of linear growth begins later, but is limited to the first nine months of life.[12]

There is good evidence that infants who are SGA because of third trimester malnutrition may be capable of catch-up growth, given adequate postnatal nutrition, whereas those who have had a more prolonged period of malnutrition or are genetically small are not.

However, a crucial issue must be whether the catch-up process, or the improved nutrition responsible for this, is important for the short- or long-term benefit of the child.

Commenting on the significance to the growth retarded infant of his extensive work on the brain growth spurt in different species including man, Dobbing has drawn attention to the fact that the

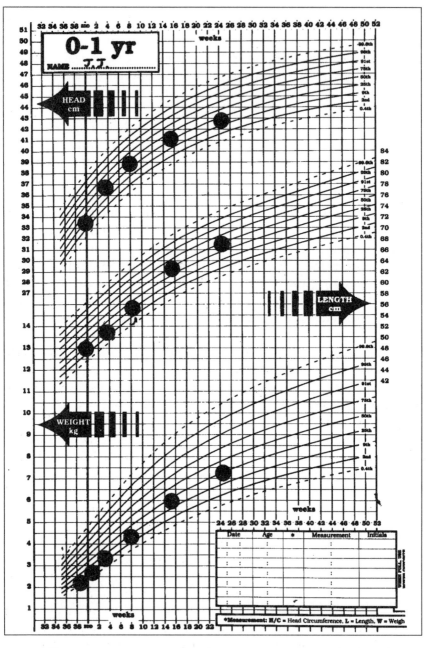

Fig. 2. *The growth chart of a male infant born at 39 weeks gestation with birth weight 2,260 g.* He demonstrated catch-up in weight, length and head circumference in the first six months of life.

prenatal period in humans represents only a small proportion of the whole of the brain growth spurt, so the IUGR infant may escape lasting brain cell deficit, provided birth truly releases him from growth constraint.[13] Continuing postnatal growth constraint, however, such that catch-up is less than adequate, may be expected to lead to poor brain growth.

Evidence that catch-up growth may be beneficial to the growth retarded infant in the medium-term is hinted at in relation to further growth and neurodevelopmental progress. Fitzhardinge and Steven reported that those children born small-for-dates whose four-year height exceeded the third percentile had shown an accelerated growth velocity in the first six months.[14]

In a study of SGA infants, in which neurological maturation as well as growth were followed over the first 12 months of life, Ounsted *et al.* found positive associations between changes in somatic measures and in neurological scores over the first six months.[15] Those infants who grew faster also matured faster neurologically during this time.

There is also some indirect evidence from studies of the fetal and infant origins of adult disease that catch-up growth may confer benefit in later life, reducing the risks of ischaemic heart disease, chronic obstructive airways disease and impaired glucose tolerance.[2]

All this information together therefore provides strong arguments to effect the best possible nutrition and optimum early postnatal growth in infants who have suffered malnutrition before birth. The enteral assimilation of nutrients must therefore occupy a key role in this, and the question inevitably arises about the state of the gastrointestinal tract in infants who have suffered prenatal undernutrition: how able is it to cope with the increased demand after birth of digesting, absorbing and utilising nutrients?

Factors that may limit catch-up growth

The gastrointestinal tract and its associated organs, in particular the pancreas, have a high rate of protein synthesis and turnover. It is not surprising, therefore, that animal and human studies have shown that malnutrition in fetal life causes abnormalities in the structure and function of the small intestine and exocrine pancreas. Suboptimal function of digestive and absorptive processes may limit the ability of the growth retarded infant to show satisfactory catch-up growth.

Intestinal effects

Animal work in three different species has shown the effects of IUGR on small intestinal structure and function. Experimentally induced IUGR in rat pups produced a decreased intestinal weight and a reduction in DNA content and in cell number.[16] Total lactase, maltase and alkaline phosphatase activities were decreased. Naturally occurring IUGR in the piglet, said to be a good model of IUGR in human infants, produced a proportionately longer but thinner-walled intestine.[17] The small intestinal surface area in IUGR piglets was reduced, and the average number of villi per unit area of small intestine and the height of the villi were also significantly reduced—all resulting in a markedly reduced area for absorption of nutrients. Similar results were found in a study of IUGR in sheep produced by maternal carunclectomy, with marked reductions in the thickness of the wall and mucosa, villus height and crypt depth, and densities of villi and crypts.[18]

Ethical considerations mean that studies of the effects of IUGR on the gastrointestinal tract in the human infant have concentrated on function rather than structure. Ducker *et al.* found that D(+)-xylose absorption, a marker of functional absorptive area of the small intestine, was lower in SGA infants than in appropriately grown infants in the first week of life.[19] The SGA group also showed the least rise in absorption over the first three weeks of life. The same workers also found a significant reduction in active D-glucose absorption in IUGR infants.[20] Macromolecular absorption in SGA infants was studied using human α-lactalbumin as a marker protein.[21] Serum α-lactalbumin concentration after a human milk feed was significantly higher in the SGA infants than in appropriately grown infants of similar gestational age, reflecting uptake across a 'leaky' mucosa. This difference was still significant at six weeks of age, suggesting that IUGR causes a delay in intestinal maturation.

Pancreatic effects

Animal studies have also provided information on the effects of intra-uterine malnutrition on exocrine pancreatic function. Lebenthal *et al.* found that growth retarded rat fetuses had reduced pancreatic weights and significantly reduced specific activities of amylase and lipase.[22] In the previously mentioned study of IUGR in pigs,[17] effects on the pancreas were also observed. The pancreas was the only organ which remained significantly smaller in the IUGR group when corrected for body weight, suggesting it to be particularly vulnerable. Functionally, the lipase activity was significantly lower in piglets with IUGR than in controls.

Duodenal juice obtained from SGA human infants showed that the lipase and trypsin activities were negatively correlated with the degree of IUGR.[23] Faecal chymotrypsin has been shown to be a reliable index of pancreatic function, with the advantages of being non-invasive and inexpensive. Faecal chymotrypsin concentrations were measured serially in pre-term infants of 32 weeks or less gestation.[24] Concentrations were significantly lower in SGA infants compared with those who were appropriately sized.

Substantial evidence has therefore emerged both from animal and from human studies that IUGR has major effects on the morphology, function and maturation of the gastrointestinal tract and pancreas. These pathophysiological events could have a significant limiting effect on catch-up growth in IUGR infants.

Optimising catch-up

Having argued that catch-up growth is important to IUGR infants for future health and development and that digestive and absorptive capacities may be impaired by intra-uterine malnutrition, what nutritional strategies can be adopted to optimise postnatal growth? The malnourished infant tends to consume more milk per unit body weight than a well-grown counterpart so it is important to allow the infant to drink *ad libitum*.[25] Breast feeding *per se* does not appear to confer any significant advantage to catch-up growth,[26] though of course it has other benefits which still make it the feeding method of choice. Increasing the protein or calorie content of the feed has been shown not to make any difference to catch-up growth.[27]

All these approaches have concentrated on the type and quantity of nutrients offered to the young growth retarded infant. One approach which has not been followed is to attempt to aid repair of the damaged gastrointestinal mucosa, and so enhance uptake of nutrients from the ingested milk. Human milk contains many substances which have growth-promoting activity on the gastrointestinal mucosa, raising the question whether supplementing infant formula with these substances could help optimise catch-up growth for those IUGR infants whose mothers are not breast feeding.

Nucleotides

Nucleotides are one group of substances that may help in this way. They are found in high concentrations in human breast milk, and over the last few years have been incorporated into infant milk formulas in Japan, the USA and Spain. Nucleotides are the building blocks of nucleic acid needed for DNA and RNA synthesis, so the highest demand for them is in organs with a high rate of cell turnover such as the gastrointestinal mucosa. Although it appears that the cells of the gastrointestinal mucosa are capable of *de novo* synthesis, this pathway may be inadequate in conditions of high demand such as recovery from malnutrition.[28] If the diet is free of nucleotides in this situation, cellular proliferation and mucosal repair will be impaired, whereas nucleotide supplementation may allow regeneration to proceed at an optimal rate. Approximately 15–30% of the total nitrogen in human milk is non-protein nitrogen and 20% of this consists of nucleotides.[29] Animal studies have shown that weanling rats fed nucleotide-free diets have shorter villi, lower maltase activity, and less protein and DNA in the jejunum.[30] Nucleoside supplementation in mice induced increased villus density and deeper crypts.[31]

Growth factors

Human milk is also rich in growth factors—low molecular weight proteins that initiate growth responses in target cells through binding to specific cell-surface receptors followed by internalisation of the entire complex into the cell. Epidermal growth factor (EGF) has been identified as the major growth factor in human milk, accounting for more than 70% of the total mitogenic activity.[32] There is virtually no EGF activity in modified cow's milk formulas. EGF has been shown in animal studies to increase DNA and protein synthesis in the gut and to accelerate maturation of brush-border enzymes in the perinatal period. The intestine appears to be more responsive to EGF following starvation, intestinal resection and total parenteral nutrition-induced villus atrophy. In these situations, EGF acts to increase the absorptive surface area.

Like nucleotides, EGF is not an essential component of infant nutrition but it may improve the efficiency of growth under conditions of poor nutrition, such as following intra-uterine malnutrition. Both nucleotides and EGF offer potential as growth-promoting agents on the atrophic gastrointestinal mucosa associated with IUGR and may aid the mucosal repair and recovery, thus optimising absorption of nutrients and possibly catch-up growth.

Conclusion

IUGR is associated with postnatal morbidity which may extend into and throughout adult life. Optimal catch-up growth would seem to be desirable, but may be impaired by associated atrophy of the small intestinal mucosa and the pancreas. Therapeutic manoeuvres which act by reversing this atrophy may improve catch-up growth, and supplementation of infant formulas with nucleotides, EGF or other growth-promoting substances may be worth exploring further.

References

1. Budin PC. *The nurseling: the feeding and hygiene of premature and full-term infants.* Translation, Moroney W, London, 1907
2. Barker DJP, ed. *Fetal and infant origins of adult disease.* London: British Medical Journal Books, 1993
3. Gruenwald P. Pathology of the deprived fetus and its supply line. *Ciba Foundation Symposia* 1974; **27**: 3–26
4. Bhargava SK, Sachdev HP, Iyer PU, Ramji S. Current status of infant growth measurements in the perinatal period in India. *Acta Paediatrica Scandinavica* 1985; **319** (Suppl): 103–10
5. King A, Loke YW. Unexplained fetal growth retardation: what is the cause? *Archives of Disease in Childhood* 1994; **70**: F225–7
6. Gardosi J, Chang A, Kalyan B, Sahota D, Symonds EM. Customised antenatal growth charts. *Lancet* 1992; **339**: 283–7
7. Fancourt R, Campbell S, Harvey D, Norman AP. Follow-up study of small-for-dates babies. *British Medical Journal* 1976; **i**: 1435–7
8. Dobbing J. The later growth of the brain and its vulnerability. In: Davis JA, Dobbing J, eds. *Scientific foundations of paediatrics,* 2nd edn. London: William Heinemann Medical Books Ltd, 1981: 744–58
9. Fitzhardinge PM, Steven EM. The small-for-date infant. II. Neurological and intellectual sequelae. *Pediatrics* 1972; **50**: 50–7
10. Prader A, Tanner JM, von Harnack GA. Catch-up growth following illness or starvation. *Journal of Pediatrics* 1963; **62**: 646–59
11. Ounsted M, Taylor ME. The postnatal growth of children who were small-for-dates or large-for-dates at birth. *Developmental Medicine and Child Neurology* 1971; **13**: 421–34
12. Fitzhardinge PM, Inwood S. Long-term growth in small-for-date children. *Acta Paediatrica Scandinavica* 1989; **349** (Suppl): 27–33
13. Dobbing J. The later growth of the brain and its vulnerability. *Pediatrics* 1975; **53**: 2–6
14. Fitzhardinge PM, Steven EM. The small-for-date infant. I. Later growth patterns. *Pediatrics* 1972; **49**: 671–81
15. Ounsted M, Moar VA, Scott A. Neurological development of small-for-gestational age babies during the first year of life. *Early Human Development* 1988; **16**: 163–72
16. Lebenthal E, Hatch T, Chrzanowski B, Krasner J, *et al.* The effect of intrauterine growth retardation (IUGR) and postnatal malnutrition on the development of intestinal brush border enzymes. *Acta Paediatrica Belgica* 1978; **31**: 169–70
17. Xu R-J, Mellor DJ, Birtles MJ, Reynolds GW, Simpson HV. Impact of intrauterine growth retardation on the gastrointestinal tract and the pancreas in newborn pigs. *Journal of Pediatric Gastroenterology and Nutrition* 1994; **18**: 231–40
18. Avila CG, Harding R, Rees S, Robinson SM. Small intestinal development in growth-retarded fetal sheep. *Journal of Pediatric Gastroenterology and Nutrition* 1989; **8**: 507–15

19. Ducker DA, Hughes CA, Warren I, McNeish AS. Neonatal gut function, measured by the one hour blood D(+) xylose test: influence of gestational age and size. *Gut* 1980; **21**: 133–6

20. McNeish AS, Ducker DA, Warren IF, Davies DP, *et al.* The influence of gestational age and size on the absorption of D-xylose and D-glucose from the small intestine of the human neonate. *Ciba Foundation Symposia* 1979; **70**: 267–79

21. Boehm G, Jakobsson I, Månsson M, Räihä NCR. Macromolecular absorption in small-for-gestational-age infants. *Acta Paediatrica* 1992; **81**: 864–7

22. Lebenthal E, Nitzan M, Chrzanowski BL, Krantz B. The effect of reduced maternofetal blood flow on the development of fetal pancreatic acinar cells and enzymes. *Pediatric Research* 1980; **14**: 1356–9

23. Boehm G, Bierbach U, Senger H, Jakobsson I, *et al.* Activities of lipase and trypsin in duodenal juice of infants small for gestational age. *Journal of Pediatric Gastroenterology and Nutrition* 1991; **12**: 324–7

24. Kolacek S, Puntis JWL, Lloyd DR, Brown GA, Booth IW. Ontogeny of pancreatic exocrine function *Archives of Disease in Childhood* 1990; **65**: 178–81

25. Ounsted M, Sleigh G. The infant's self-regulation of food intake and weight gain. *Lancet* 1975; **i**: 1393–7

26. Davies DP. Infant's self-regulation of food intake [letter]. *Lancet* 1975; **ii**: 366–7

27. Davies DP. Growth of 'small-for-dates' babies. *Early Human Development* 1981; **5**: 95–105

28. Savaiano DA, Clifford AJ. Adenine, the precursor of nucleic acids in intestinal cells unable to synthesize purines *de novo*. *Journal of Nutrition* 1981; **111**: 1816–22

29. Janas LM, Picciano MF. The nucleotide profile of human milk. *Pediatric Research* 1982; **16**: 659–62

30. Uauy R, Stringel G, Thomas R, Quan R. Effect of dietary nucleosides on growth and maturation of the developing gut in the rat. *Journal of Pediatric Gastroenterology and Nutrition* 1990; **10**: 497–503

31. Quan R, Barness LA, Uauy R. Do infants need nucleotide supplemented formula for optimal nutrition? *Journal of Pediatric Gastroenterology and Nutrition* 1990; **11**: 429–34

32. Read LC. Milk growth factors. In: Cockburn F, ed. *Fetal and neonatal growth*. Chichester: John Wiley & Sons Ltd, 1988: 131–52

9 | Nutrition in the sick neonate

John Puntis
Senior Lecturer in Paediatrics and Child Health, University of Leeds; Consultant Paediatrician, Peter Congdon Neonatal Unit, The General Infirmary at Leeds

The outlook both for prematurely born infants[1] and for those requiring major surgery in the newborn period[2] has steadily improved over the past two decades. This is a result of advances in many different areas of neonatal intensive care, including nutritional support. However, the inability to reproduce intra-uterine growth rates in the pre-term infant is only one example of the reality that many fundamental questions regarding their nutrition remain unanswered. Only recently have epidemiological studies indicated the probability of long-term consequences of poor nutrition during early life.[3] The particular implications for the sick neonate remain a matter for speculation and concern.

The problems of undernutrition in adult hospital patients have recently been highlighted,[4] with attention focused on how malnutrition as a multisystem disorder contributes to morbidity and mortality in a wide range of conditions. The nutritional needs of the newborn infant are unique; when the energy demands of critical illness compete with requirements for growth and development in a baby with little or no reserves, the provision of nutritional support is an urgent priority. For example, a small pre-term infant of 1 kg, who has perhaps no more than 10 g of storage fat, might survive only four days if starved, a 2 kg baby 12 days, and a 3.5 kg term infant 32 days.[5] Many infants now surviving neonatal intensive care are well below 1 kg at birth. Whether the enteral or parenteral route is used for nutrition depends chiefly on gestational age and clinical state, but a strict dichotomy is often inappropriate since each approach can complement the other.

Parenteral nutrition

Maintaining growth during long-term parenteral nutrition (PN) in an infant with a short bowel was first reported in 1968.[6] The prospects for newborn babies requiring gastrointestinal surgery were so radically transformed by this new treatment that prospective studies comparing PN with conventional management were considered unnecessary. With increasingly widespread use of PN, its usefulness for pre-term infants with an intact but immature gastrointestinal tract seemed self evident. However, the paucity of clinical trials comparing enteral nutrition (EN) and PN in this group makes evaluation of its benefits difficult. Overall, it seems likely that PN has contributed to increasing survival amongst ever smaller and more immature infants, but at least one study has suggested an increased mortality and higher risk of poor growth, nosocomial infection and chronic lung disease associated with PN.[7] There remains considerable variation in its use between different units, reflecting lack of agreement regarding precise indications.

Small bowel failure secondary to congenital/acquired abnormality of the gastrointestinal tract is an absolute indication for PN, together with necrotising enterocolitis (NEC) where cessation of enteral feeding is a universally accepted principle of management. Respiratory failure requiring ventilation, 'immaturity' of the digestive system, and prevention of NEC may be regarded as relative indications where there is room for considerable debate. Decisions regarding the use of PN are also influenced by local perceptions of safety and efficacy. For example, units with a high incidence of central venous catheter sepsis may (rightly) favour EN over PN.[8]

Parenteral nutrition regimens

Although there is some general measure of agreement about energy and nutrient requirements, the needs of the sick infant are difficult to assess. Nutritional inadequacies are important contributory factors to the early growth failure regularly found in survivors of neonatal intensive care.[9] Energy is usually provided as a combination of glucose and lipid, and should be sufficient to prevent gluconeogenesis and breakdown of lean body mass as well as providing for growth and organ development. Traditionally, PN has been started slowly once the infant is considered 'stable', and then gradually built up over a week or more. However, the recognition that such caution is probably unwarranted—since illness and surgery rapidly lead to negative nitrogen balance—has prompted the introduction of accelerated feeding schedules.[10,11]

Carbohydrate. Initial infusion rates of 5–6 mg/kg/min will maintain normoglycaemia. Intake can be increased to 14–16 g/kg/day over several days, and further increased—if tolerated—when weight gain is suboptimal. Glucose intolerance is sometimes seen in the extremely low birth weight infant or during episodes of sepsis. In the latter condition, temporary reduction of carbohydrate supply is all that is required, but in the tiny infant insulin infusion may be necessary to achieve an adequate calorie intake.[12] Thrombophlebitis and difficulty maintaining peripheral venous access can be important contributors to poor nutrition, and the central route is a more reliable way to deliver PN. A central venous catheter allows high glucose concentrations to be given safely, particularly in the fluid-restricted infant.

Nitrogen. Nitrogen is supplied as synthetic crystalline L-amino acids. The ideal composition of solutions and the exact nitrogen requirements for the newborn have not been established. Histidine, tyrosine and cysteine are essential. Recognition of a taurine deficiency state[13] has led recently to incorporation of taurine in amino acid preparations. The recommended intake is about 2.5 g amino acids/kg/day, and should be given with 24–32 non-nitrogen calories/g amino acid for optimal utilisation. Abnormal plasma amino acid profiles are frequently seen during PN. Concern about high levels of aromatic amino acids has prompted a reduction in their concentration in solution.[14]

Fat. Lipid emulsions, providing essential fatty acids, are calorie-dense and isotonic. In adult patients, a combination of glucose and fat for supplying energy leads to improved protein synthesis and less water retention,[15] reduced energy expenditure,[16] and less hepatic fat infiltration. The emulsion droplets are similar in size to natural chylomicrons, and the triglyceride portion is hydrolysed by lipoprotein lipase in endothelial cells. Prematurity and growth retardation are associated with decreased lipid tolerance. Up to 2–4 g/kg/day of fat may be given, but fat clearance, particularly at higher intakes, should be monitored by measuring plasma triglycerides. There are several concerns with the use of long-chain triglyceride lipid emulsions in the sick neonate, including:

- adverse effects on oxygenation and immune function;
- formation of lipid emboli; and
- displacement of protein-bound bilirubin (with the risk of kernicterus).

Fat infusion in pre-term infants during the first week of life has been associated with a fall in arterial oxygen tension[17] and increased pulmonary vascular resistance,[18] the suggested mechanism being production of vasoactive prostaglandin metabolites of linoleic acid, the principal fatty acid in long-chain triglyceride emulsions. An increase in vasodilating prostaglandins causes unblocking of hypoxic vasoconstriction in underventilated areas of the lung. However, the magnitude of this effect is probably unimportant except in those infants with borderline hypoxaemia or with pulmonary hypertension from other causes, conditions where caution with lipid seems justified. Necropsy findings of lipid emboli in the pulmonary vasculature have also suggested a possible adverse effect of lipid emulsion on the lung. These findings almost certainly represent ante-mortem coalescence of lipid emulsion,[19] but their clinical importance is unclear.

Many studies have suggested an adverse influence of lipid on immune function. Although few have pointed to a clinically relevant effect,[20] one study of pre-term infants[21] found a 5.8-fold increase in coagulase-negative staphylococcal infection associated with Intralipid (Kabi Pharmacia). During episodes of overwhelming sepsis it is reasonable to stop lipid administration until there are signs of improvement. However, malnutrition as a result of inadequate energy intake has itself an adverse effect on immunity, and part of the response to stress includes an increase in lipolysis and a decrease in glucose utilisation. Too low a threshold for withholding lipid infusion may therefore not be without disadvantages.

Free fatty acids produced by triglyceride metabolism might theoretically displace bilirubin from albumin-binding sites and increase the risk of kernicterus, particularly in the small, sick infant. The concentration of free fatty acids likely to produce this effect *in vivo* is unknown, although it could occur when the free fatty acid/albumin ratio exceeds 6.[22] More recent studies have failed to show an effect of different rates of lipid infusion on total and apparent unbound bilirubin.[23] Until more information is available it seems prudent to limit lipid intake in pre-term infants with unconjugated hyperbilirubinaemia above 170 μmol/l.

Vitamins and trace elements. Precise needs for vitamins and trace elements remain in doubt for the pre-term infant or sick neonate.[24] Multivitamin and trace element preparations are available and provide nutrients for which deficiency states have been demonstrated (usually in adults) during long-term PN:

- the intake of zinc and copper may be inadequate, particularly during rapid growth or with diarrhoeal or ileostomy losses;

- selenium has only recently been added to trace element preparations;

- accumulation of aluminium, which contaminates many PN products, has been reported in the bones of pre-term infants given intravenous fluids[25] and can occasionally accumulate sufficiently to cause encephalopathy;
- manganese is excreted in the bile and may accumulate in patients with cholestasis, causing damage to the basal ganglia and probably further damaging the liver. This finding has demonstrated the need to re-evaluate manganese intake and monitor plasma levels in infants with hepatic dysfunction.

Prescribing and monitoring parenteral nutrition

The following should be taken into account in prescribing PN for the sick newborn:

- fluid retention or excess loss;
- electrolyte losses in nasogastric aspirate, urine or stomas;
- organ failure;
- glucose intolerance;
- additional intravenous infusions and line flushes;
- partial enteral feeds;
- sepsis;
- jaundice; and
- route of venous access.

In practice, it is simpler to perform the necessary calculations using a computer programme designed for formulating PN.[26] Such a system:

- allows individualisation of prescription;
- reduces wastage of PN components;
- facilitates maintenance of fluid and electrolyte homoeostasis; and
- improves communication with the pharmacy.

PN infusion rarely leads to unexpected and serious biochemical derangement in the stable surgical infant,[27] although glucose tolerance should always be closely monitored and fat clearance can be reliably assessed only by measuring plasma triglycerides.[28] Frequent biochemical monitoring is usually undertaken in the unstable or sick neonate, irrespective of PN.

Enteral nutrition

Enteral feeding has several potential advantages in addition to its simplicity and low cost. For example, it provides glutamine, an essential respiratory fuel for cells of the gastrointestinal tract;[29] this may help to maintain mucosal integrity and immunological function, decreasing the risk of bacterial translocation. PN may offer no clear advantage in the sick neonate whose gut is functioning unless fluid restriction prevents full-volume feeds. A common problem in the pre-term newborn, however, is functional immaturity of the gastrointestinal tract, in particular with poor gut motility (often compounded by hypoxia, hypotension or sepsis), making it impossible to achieve an adequate enteral nutritional intake during the most critical period of early illness.

By 22–28 weeks gestation, morphology of the fetal small intestinal mucosa resembles that of the adult and the activity of many digestive enzymes has almost reached adult values, although liver, biliary, pancreatic and motor function are less well developed. Hazards of milk feeds may have been overestimated. For example, a survey of regional neonatal units in the UK found that about one-third rarely use enteral feeds during mechanical ventilation for fear of aspiration[30]—which was thought likely to occur secondary to poor oesophageal peristalsis and underdevelopment of the gastro-oesophageal sphincter mechanism. However, when reflux was studied in a group of nine pre-term infants, the gastro-oesophageal pressure gradient was found to be reduced by mechanical ventilation (probably related to the use of positive end expiratory pressure), suggesting that reflux is less likely to occur during ventilation than during spontaneous respiration.[30]

An investigation of the motor response of the small intestine to enteral feeds in pre-term infants showed this to be dependent on the bolus volume of feed and the number of days on which enteral feeds had been given.[31] The post-conceptional age of the infant does not seem to be important, implying that the early introduction of enteral nutrition enhances the motor response of the small intestine to feeds. Other aspects of gastrointestinal function may also be influenced by enteral feeding. For example, although the activity of mucosal lactase is low in the fetus of 26–30 weeks gestation, clinical lactose intolerance appears uncommon in the pre-term infant. Measurement of disaccharidase activity in small bowel juice (which is highly correlated with mucosal enzyme activity) from 26–29 weeks gestation infants fed human milk showed lactase activity within the reference range for older infants and children.[32] These adaptive changes in the bowel may be mediated through gut hormones whose release is considerably reduced in patients given only PN.[33] Priming the gastrointestinal tract with low volumes of milk before full enteral feeding is started has been shown to improve feeding tolerance and lead to a more rapid increase in serum gastrin concentration.[34]

Necrotising enterocolitis

The great majority of infants who develop NEC have been enterally fed but debate continues about the precise importance of milk feeds as a risk factor. A matched case-control study of 59 infants with NEC implicated both early feeding and large increments in the pathogenesis of the disease.[35] Some units have reported a decreased incidence of NEC associated with a change to later introduction of enteral nutrition, but historical case comparisons are unreliable—particularly when the incidence of NEC is variable. Small randomised prospective trials have suggested that PN merely postpones the onset of NEC[36] and that early enteral feeding does not affect the incidence. When enteral feeds are given, breast milk seems to have an important protective effect.[37]

Conclusion

Adequate nutritional support is an urgent priority in the sick newborn infant with limited energy reserves. Small intestinal failure secondary to congenital or acquired gastrointestinal disease is an absolute indication for PN, but PN is expensive and complex when compared to enteral nutrition and associated with a number of different hazards. Although it seems likely that widespread use of PN in the sick pre-term infant with functional immaturity of the bowel has contributed to improved survival, good data to support this contention are lacking. When immaturity precludes full enteral feeding, small volumes of milk to prime the gut may lead to more rapid maturation of the gastrointestinal tract.[38,39]

References

1. Cooke RWI. Outcome and costs of care for the very immature infant. *British Medical Bulletin* 1988; **44**: 1133–51
2. Goulet OJ, Revillon Y, Jan D, De Potter S, *et al.* Neonatal short bowel syndrome. *Journal of Pediatrics* 1991; **119**: 18–23
3. Barker DJP. The foetal and infant origins of inequalities in health in Britain. *Journal of Public Health Medicine* 1991; **13**: 64–8
4. Lennard-Jones JE, ed. *A positive approach to nutrition as treatment.* King's Fund Report. London: King's Fund Centre, 1992
5. Heird WC, Driscoll JM, Schulinger JN, Grebin B, Winters RW. Intravenous alimentation in pediatric patients. *Journal of Pediatrics* 1972; **80**: 351–72

6. Wilmore DW, Dudrick SJ. Growth and development of an infant receiving all nutrients by vein. *Journal of the American Medical Association* 1968; **203**: 860–4

7. Unger A, Goetzman BW, Chan C, Lyons AB, Miller MF. Nutritional practices and outcome of extremely premature infants. *American Journal of Diseases of Children* 1986; **140**: 1027–33

8. Glass J, Hume R, Lang MA, Forfar JO. Parenteral nutrition compared with transpyloric feeding. *Archives of Disease in Childhood* 1984; **59**: 131–5

9. Georgieff MK, Hoffman JS, Pereira GR, Bernbaum J, Hoffman-Williamson M. Effect of neonatal caloric deprivation on head growth and 1-year developmental status in preterm infants. *Journal of Pediatrics* 1985; **107**: 581–7

10. Saini J, MacMahon P, Morgan JB, Kovar IZ. Early parenteral feeding of amino acids. *Archives of Disease in Childhood* 1989; **64**: 1362–6

11. Gilbertson N, Kovar IZ, Cox DJ, Crowe L, Palmer NT. Introduction of intravenous lipid administration on the first day of life. *Journal of Pediatrics* 1991; **119**: 615–23

12. Binder ND, Raschko PK, Benda GI, Reynolds JW. Insulin infusion with parenteral nutrition in extremely low birth weight infants with hyperglycaemia. *Journal of Pediatrics* 1989; **114**: 273–80

13. Geggel HS, Ament ME, Heckenlively JR, Martin DA, Kopple JD. Nutritional requirement for taurine in patients receiving long term parenteral nutrition. *New England Journal of Medicine* 1985; **312**: 142–6

14. Puntis JWL, Ball PA, Preece MA, Green A, *et al.* Egg and breast milk based nitrogen sources compared. *Archives of Disease in Childhood* 1989; **64**: 1472–7

15. Macfie J, Smith RC, Hill GL. Glucose or fat as a nonprotein energy source? A controlled clinical trial in gastroenterological patients requiring intravenous nutrition. *Gastroenterology* 1981; **80**: 103–7

16. Macfie J, Holmfield JH, King RF, Hill GL. Effect of the energy source on changes in energy expenditure and respiratory quotient during total parenteral nutrition. *Journal of Parenteral and Enteral Nutrition* 1983; **7**: 1–5

17. Pereira GR, Fox WW, Stanley CA, Baker L, Schwartz JG. Decreased oxygenation and hyperlipidemia during intravenous fat infusions in premature infants. *Pediatrics* 1980; **66**: 26–30

18. Lloyd TR, Boucek MM. Effect of Intralipid on the neonatal pulmonary bed: an echographic study. *Journal of Pediatrics* 1986; **108**: 130–3

19. Puntis JWL, Rushton DI. Pulmonary intravascular lipid in neonatal necropsy specimens. *Archives of Disease in Childhood* 1991; **66**: 776–9

20. Palmblad J. Intravenous lipid emulsions and host defence—a critical review. *Clinical Nutrition* 1991; **10**: 303–8

21. Freeman J, Goldmann DA, Smith NE, Sidebottom DG, *et al.* Association of intravenous lipid emulsion and coagulase-negative staphylococcal bacteremia in neonatal intensive care units. *New England Journal of Medicine* 1990; **323**: 301–8

22. Andrew G, Chan G, Schiff D. Lipid metabolism in the neonate. 1. The effects of Intralipid infusion on plasma triglyceride and free fatty acid concentrations in the neonate. *Journal of Pediatrics* 1976; **88**: 273–8

23. Brans YW, Ritter DA, Kenny JD, Andrew DS, *et al.* Influence of intravenous fat emulsion on serum bilirubin in very low birthweight neonates. *Archives of Disease in Childhood* 1987; **62**: 156–60

24. Greene HL, Hambidge KM, Schanler R, Tsang RC. Guidelines for the use of vitamins, trace elements, calcium, magnesium and phosphorus in infants and children receiving total parenteral nutrition. Report of the Subcommittee on Pediatric Parenteral Nutrient Requirements from the Committee on Clinical Practice Issues of The American Society for Clinical Nutrition. *American Journal of Clinical Nutrition* 1988; **48**: 1324–42

25. Sedman AB, Klein GL, Merritt RJ, Miller NL, *et al.* Evidence of aluminum loading in infants receiving intravenous therapy. *New England Journal of Medicine* 1985; **312**: 1337–43

26. Ball PA, Candy DCA, Puntis JWL, McNeish AS. Portable bedside microcomputer system for management of parenteral nutrition in all age groups. *Archives of Disease in Childhood* 1985; **60**: 435–9

27. Puntis JWL, Hall SK, Green A, Smith DE, *et al.* Biochemical stability during parenteral nutrition in children. *Clinical Nutrition* 1993; **12**: 153–9

28. Schreiner RL, Glick MR, Nordschow CD, Gresham EL. An evaluation of methods to monitor infants receiving intravenous lipids. *Journal of Pediatrics* 1979; **94**: 197–200

29. Lacey JM, Wilmore DW. Is glutamine a conditionally essential amino acid? *Nutrition Reviews* 1990; **48**: 297–309

30. Newell SJ, Morgan MEI, Durbin GM, Booth IW, McNeish AS. Does mechanical ventilation precipitate gastro-oesophageal reflux during enteral feeding? *Archives of Disease in Childhood* 1989; **64**: 1352–5

31. Bisset WM, Watt J, Rivers RPA, Milla PJ. Postprandial motor response of the small intestine to enteral feeds in preterm infants. *Archives of Disease in Childhood* 1989; **64**: 1356–61

32. Mayne AJ, Brown GA, Sule D, McNeish AS. Postnatal development of disaccharidase activities in jejunal fluid of preterm neonates. *Gut* 1986; **27**: 1357–61

33. Lucas A, Bloom SR, Aynsley-Green A. Metabolic and endocrine effects of depriving preterm infants of enteral nutrition. *Acta Paediatrica Scandinavica* 1983; **72**: 245–9

34. Meetze WH, Valentine C, McGuigan JE, Conlon M, *et al.* Gastrointestinal priming prior to full enteral nutrition in very low birthweight infants. *Journal of Pediatric Gastroenterology and Nutrition* 1992; **15**: 163–70

35. McKeown RE, Marsh TD, Amarnath U, Garrison CZ, *et al.* Role of delayed feeding and of feeding increments in necrotizing enterocolitis. *Journal of Pediatrics* 1992; **121**: 764–70

36. LaGamma EF, Ostertag SG, Birenbaum H. Failure of delayed oral feedings to prevent necrotizing enterocolitis. *American Journal of Diseases of Children* 1985; **139**: 385–9

37. Lucas A, Cole TJ. Breast milk and neonatal necrotising enterocolitis. *Lancet* 1991; **336**: 1519–23

38. Dunn L, Hulman S, Weiner J, Kliegman R. Beneficial effects of early hypocaloric enteral feeding on neonatal gastrointestinal function: preliminary report of a randomized trial. *Journal of Pediatrics* 1988; **112**: 622–9

39. Slagle TA, Gross SJ. Effect of early low-volume enteral substrate on subsequent feeding tolerance in very low birthweight infants. *Journal of Pediatrics* 1988; **113**: 526–31

PART THREE

Nutrition for the sick and problem child

10 | The nutritional management of gastrointestinal disease in childhood

Ian W Booth

Professor of Paediatric Gastroenterology and Nutrition, University of Birmingham, Institute of Child Health, Birmingham

The gut has enormous reserve capacity, and its adaptive responses can mask even quite marked functional defects resulting from disease. However, nutrient absorption and assimilation are such key features of normal gastrointestinal function that malnutrition and impaired growth are early features of diffuse gut and liver pathology. Assessment of nutritional status and manipulation of nutrient intake therefore play an essential role in the management of gastrointestinal and hepatic disease. Dietary manipulation also has an important and recently recognised primary role in the specific circumstances of the induction of remission in Crohn's disease and in the enhancement of the adaptive response following massive small intestinal resection.

Key points

A number of key points should be borne in mind when planning the nutritional management of children with gastrointestinal disease (Table 1).

- *Pathophysiology should define treatment*

A working knowledge of the pathophysiology of the disease process is essential to rational management. This implies that as accurate a diagnosis as possible is required. 'Malabsorption' is no longer an acceptable end-point. For example, the osmotic diarrhoea which characterises sucrase-isomaltase deficiency and secondary lactose intolerance following gastroenteritis have many superficial similarities, but each requires a quite distinct dietary approach. Similarly, correction of the profound malnutrition which is such a frequent feature of severe prolonged cholestasis requires a knowledge of the

Table 1. Key points in the nutritional management of gastrointestinal and liver disease in children

---

- a precise knowledge of the pathophysiology of disease is essential in providing rational nutritional management
- use the gut whenever possible, even if the amounts of nutrient tolerated are nutritionally insignificant; a trophic effect is still likely to be present
- malnutrition damages the gut
- nutritional care needs a multidisciplinary approach

---

physiology of luminal triglyceride hydrolysis solubilisation and absorption.

- *Use the gut whenever possible*

Parenteral nutrition is important in restoring normal nutritional status in children with intestinal failure, but *total* parenteral nutrition induces functional and structural atrophy in the gut. Residual absorptive function should therefore be used whenever possible. To obtain maximal absorption, the gut must function throughout the entire 24 hours, which implies that the nutrients will be delivered by continuous infusion through a nasogastric tube or feeding gastrostomy. The trophic effects of luminal nutrients are such that their continued administration is usually indicated, even in nutritionally insignificant amounts.

- *Malnutrition damages the gut*

The effects of severe protein-energy malnutrition in a multisystem disorder include impaired immune status, depressed mood, impaired wound healing and reduced skeletal muscle and myocardial function. However, the major impact is felt by the gut and virtually every feature of gastrointestinal disorder may result. For example, gastric acid secretion, pancreatic exocrine function, small intestinal enterocyte function and colonic electrolyte absorption are all reduced. Nutritional repletion therefore has an important role in its own right. The ability of the gut to self-repair will be impaired until this takes place, and it represents an important indication for parenteral nutrition.

- *Nutritional care requires a team approach*

The needs of the malnourished child with gastrointestinal disease cut across many different professional disciplines. Cooperation and pooling of expertise among those involved in the care of such children offer the greatest opportunity for more rational, safe and effective provision of nutritional support.

Indications for nutritional support

PRIMARY THERAPY

Induction of remission in Crohn's disease (Table 2)

Crohn's disease is a full-thickness, diffuse, chronic inflammatory disorder, potentially affecting any part of the gut from the mouth to the anus. It is of unknown cause, and therefore curative treatment is not available. Malnutrition and anorexia are common. One-third of affected adolescents experience growth failure and pubertal delay.

At present, no intervention has been shown to prevent relapse and thereby alter the natural history of the disease. Until recently, corticosteroids were the mainstay of treatment for inducing remission of active disease. Unfortunately, steroids have many well-recognised side-effects. In Crohn's disease in particular, many adolescents find the cushingoid appearance unacceptable, and steroids tend to suppress rather than enhance growth.

It was shown in adults in the 1980s that the administration of an elemental diet as the sole means of nutrition for six weeks was as effective as oral prednisolone in inducing remission. In general, about 80% of patients went into remission on either treatment. There were a number of advantages associated with the administration of an elemental diet, including a greater improvement in haemoglobin and serum albumin. Subsequently, a similar effect was seen in children, with the additional benefit that those patients who went into remission in response to an elemental diet showed catch-

Table 2. Induction of remission in Crohn's disease: enteral elemental diet compared with steroids

---

Enteral nutrition:

- at least as effective as steroids in inducing remission
- better growth and nutrition response
- variable duration of remission, according to site of disease
- preferred choice in small intestinal disease
- mechanisms of action unknown

---

up growth in the six months following treatment, whereas the steroid-treated group continued to experience growth failure.

An elemental, chemically defined diet (Elemental 028, Scientific Hospital Supplies) in which nitrogen is provided as crystalline amino acids is now the treatment of choice of most paediatric gastroenterologists. About half my patients elect to drink E028, and half prefer to have a nasogastric tube.

One area of uncertainty has been the duration of remission achieved with an elemental diet compared with steroids. This has recently been examined in an analysis of patients treated at the Children's Hospital. Because of the well-recognised benefits of an elemental diet with respect to growth, it was felt inappropriate to embark on a randomised trial; instead, patients treated with an elemental diet were compared with historic controls who received steroids. The results confirmed that E028 was at least as good as prednisolone in inducing remission, and that growth in the 12 months after stopping the elemental diet was significantly better than in the steroid-treated group (Figure 1). Although the groups became small when stratified for disease site, those patients with

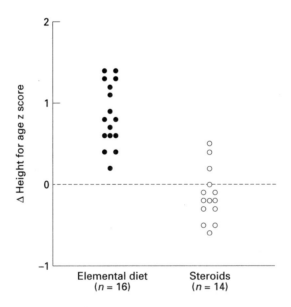

Fig. 1. *Growth in children with Crohn's disease following induction of remission with either an elemental diet or oral prednisolone* (z-score is the standard deviation score—the number of standard deviations an observation is above or below the mean) (see Further reading no. 3).

small bowel disease treated with an elemental diet had a substantially longer remission than those treated with steroids; when the colon was affected, the reverse tended to be true—remission on the elemental diet was shorter, and steroids had a small benefit. Thus, an elemental diet has clear advantages in small bowel intestinal Crohn's disease. The somewhat larger remission associated with steroids in colonic disease has to be balanced against the poorer growth seen in patients who receive prednisolone.

It is not known why an elemental diet is effective. A reduction in antigen load, lower luminal residue and alteration in bacterial flora have all been implicated. Recent evidence suggests that a polymeric diet (one containing whole protein) may be just as effective as an elemental diet. If confirmed, this would circumvent one of the major problems of an elemental diet—its marked unpalatability.

Enhancing the adaptive response in short bowel syndrome

Short bowel syndrome is a relatively common problem in neonatal surgical units. The disorder arises following massive resection for necrotising enterocolitis, or as a result of congenital anomalies such as intestinal atresia or gastroschisis. Although 90% of affected neonates now survive without the need for long-term parenteral nutrition at home, the need for it in hospital may last for many months and some children die of liver failure secondary to parenteral nutrition-induced liver disease.

Following massive small intestinal resection the remaining gut undergoes a process of adaptation, whereby functional and structural hypertrophy take place which eventually supports sufficient absorptive function to permit survival without parenteral nutrition. This adaptive response is driven by a wide variety of agents, but the presence of luminal nutrients appears to be the most important single factor. Recent evidence in experimental animals suggests that the administration of certain nutrients may accelerate this process:

1. *Pectin.* Strictly speaking, pectin is not a nutrient but a water-soluble, non-starch polysaccharide which escapes digestion in the small intestine and is completely fermented to short-chain fatty acids in the colon. It has little effect on faecal bulk in man, in contrast to other forms of fibre. Addition of pectin to food delays gastric emptying and slows transit through the human small intestine. It has a trophic effect in the colon, where short-chain fatty acids are the preferred nutrient substrate of colonic sites and, rather surprisingly, a similar effect in the small intestine.

Addition of pectin to the feed of rats who have undergone 80% small intestinal resection enhances the adaptive response both in the intestine and in the pancreas. Two weeks after resection, pectin-treated animals had jejunal, ileal and colonic evidence of an enhanced weight/length ratio, increased mucosal DNA, RNA and protein content, and in the ileum there were smaller villi and deeper crypts. These effects are probably related in part to an increase in transit time, prolonged mucosal contact, and enhanced pancreatic secretion (an additional trophic factor). Luminal short-chain fatty acids also have a direct trophic effect in the colon and increase gut blood flow.

As a consequence of these impressive observations in experimental animals and preliminary studies in human short bowel syndrome, at the Children's Hospital 1% pectin is often added to the enteral feeds of patients with short bowel syndrome who do not have concurrent severe bacterial overgrowth in the small intestine. It is not possible to envisage ever having a randomised control trial of pectin in this disorder, and practice in man will continue to be dependent upon observations in experimental animals.

2. *Glutamine.* Glutamine is the preferred oxidative substrate of small intestinal enterocytes. In some studies, similar results have been found with glutamine as with pectin in animals with short gut syndrome, but not all work in experimental animals substantiates this. It is claimed that provision of 25% of the amino acids in a feed as glutamine leads to jejunal and ileal hyperplasia (even on a hypocaloric intake), enhanced weight gain, and prevention of pancreatic atrophy and of fatty change in the liver.

Similar studies in man are awaited, but a trial of glutamine supplementation of enteral feeds is appropriate in infants with severe short bowel syndrome who are failing to adapt satisfactorily to enteral feeds.

INTESTINAL FAILURE

Nutritional support by the parenteral route is essential to the survival of patients with intestinal failure. This is an uncommon problem and referral to a specialist centre with a nutritional care team is crucial. A detailed description of the management is beyond the scope of this review, but adherence to the key points outlined above and in Table 1 is particularly important in the management of this disorder. Causes of short bowel syndrome are shown in Table 3.

Most patients will experience pan-malabsorption and, to achieve maximal use of residual absorptive function, enteral feeds must be

Table 3. Causes of intestinal failure

- **short gut**
- **mucosal disease:**

—necrotising enterocolitis   —'post-gastroenteritis syndrome'

—microvillus inclusion disease   —radiation/cytotoxic enteropathy

—autoimmune enterocolitis   —HIV infection

- **pseudo-obstruction**

tailored to the individual needs of the patient. Consequently, a modular feed, in which the individual feed components can be separately manipulated, is usually required rather than a commercial formula. In general, the concentrations of carbohydrate (usually given as a glucose polymer/sucrose) and lipid (long-chain triglyceride) are increased individually to the limit of tolerance. For carbohydrate, an increase in stool volume with positive reducing substances on Clinitest signals the onset of intolerance. Serial measures of stool steatocrit have been shown to be useful in the early detection of lipid intolerance. In common with other paediatric gastroenterologists, comminuted chicken (Cow & Gate Nutricia) is our first choice of nitrogen source. These feeds are not for occasional use and an experienced dietitian is essential in their provision.

LIVER DISEASE

Severe malnutrition affects 50% of children with established cirrhosis. In children with less advanced liver disease, arm anthropometry becomes abnormal before reduction in weight and height. The early reduction in muscle and fat which is characteristic of protein-energy malnutrition in liver disease may relate to peripheral oxidation of muscle, fat malabsorption and preferential improvement of fat as an energy substrate. The precise mechanisms leading to malnutrition in liver disease are poorly understood. Clearly, anorexia and fat maldigestion are major problems; in adults, abnormal gluconeogenesis leads to reduced glycogen stores, hypoglycaemia and early recruitment of fat as an energy substrate. Nitrogen metabolism is also disturbed. In addition, portal hypertension is associated with an enteropathy and ascites which may cause food intolerance and exacerbation of protein-energy malnutrition.

Strategies for nutritional support in liver disease

1. *Increased energy intake.* Resting energy requirements in children with liver disease are increased, and the metabolic costs of sepsis and fat malabsorption further increase energy requirements. An increase in energy intake to 140–200% of the recommended daily allowance is often required; this is achieved in infants by supplementing feeds with extra fat (up to 8 g/kg/day) and carbohydrate (up to 15–20 g/kg/day).

2. *Nasogastric tube feeding.* Despite a good appetite initially, most infants and children become anorexic after a few months and need nasogastric tube feeding. This approach is effective in reversing protein-energy malnutrition and may induce a transformation in the child's mood, such that voluntary oral intake also improves. Long-term behavioural problems associated with tube feeding can be minimised if feeding is given overnight, allowing normal oral intake during the day. Gastrostomy feeding is avoided because of complications related to ascites and possible surgical problems of access to the abdominal cavity during a subsequent liver transplant procedure.

Important components of an enteral feed

1. *Fat.* Medium-chain triglycerides should be substituted for 50–70% of the long-chain triglycerides. They are more soluble and do not require lipolysis or solubilisation by luminal bile acids for absorption.

2. *Essential fatty acids.* The requirements for linoleic and linolenic acid in children with liver disease are not accurately known. The risk of deficiency is increased by jaundice, protein-energy malnutrition, and when intake of essential fatty acids is less than 500 mg/kg/day. A ratio of linoleic to linolenic acid of 5:1 is recommended because this is close to the ratio observed in breast milk.

3. *Fat-soluble vitamins.* Proprietary multivitamin preparations are inadequate. Up to 20 times the recommended daily amount of fat-soluble vitamins may be needed to produce therapeutic plasma concentrations of vitamin A and E and to prevent the occurrence of rickets and a prolonged prothrombin time (eg 5,000–20,000 units of vitamin A, 100–800 mg of vitamin E, 50–150 µg/kg of alpha-calcidol, and 5–10 mg of vitamin K daily).

4. *Carbohydrate.* A glucose polymer is used to minimise osmolality in the feed while maintaining a high energy density.

5. *Protein.* Up to 4 g/kg/day of protein may be tolerated by children with advanced liver disease without precipitation of encephalopathy. A whole-protein source is preferred because of its therapeutic effect on the gut and its palatability. The role of branched chain amino acids, which undergo extrahepatic metabolism, is still not clearly defined.

Commercially available feeds

Pregestimil (Bristol-Myers) and Pepti-Junior (Cow & Gate Nutricia) are frequently used when nutritional support is first required as they provide 40–50% medium-chain triglyceride in a nutritionally complete formula. A formula (Caprilon formula, Cow & Gate Nutricia) in which 75% of the fat is present as medium-chain triglyceride has recently become available.

Modular feeds and parenteral nutrition

In advanced liver disease, use of a modular feed is often essential. Parenteral nutrition is occasionally required for a child with end-stage liver disease when enteral feeds or infection precipitate protracted diarrhoea. Parenteral nutrition may improve encephalopathy but is usually regarded as an indication for liver transplantation.

Role of a nutritional care team (Table 4)

The benefits of a multidisciplinary nutritional care team are well-documented (Table 5). Although cost saving is perhaps not the most important aspect of a team's work, it remains an important consideration in times of increasing financial stringency. At the Children's Hospital, work carried out by clinical nurse specialists led to a sixfold reduction in catheter sepsis, leading to a cost saving of about £100,000 per annum, in addition to obvious patient

Table 4. The role of a nutritional care team

• early identification of 'at-risk' patients	• audit
• nutritional assessment	• teaching
• provision of specialised nutritional support	• research
• clinical and biochemical monitoring	

Table 5. Reported benefits of a nutritional care team

Reduction in:

- central venous catheter sepsis
- mechanical catheter complications
- metabolic complications of parenteral nutrition
- average length of course of parenteral nutrition
- expenditure of parenteral nutrition

Increase in:

- use of enteral instead of parenteral nutrition

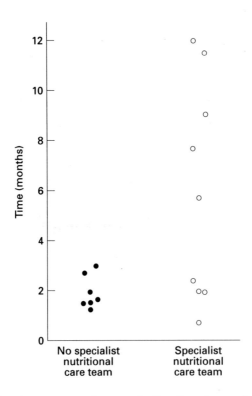

Fig. 2. *Mean time between central venous feeding line changes in children referred for assessment for small bowel transplantation.* Lines in children referred from a centre without a specialist nutritional care team had a significantly shorter life than lines in children from centres with such a team ($p < 0.02$) (see Further reading no. 4).

benefits. Providing clinical nurse specialists is therefore a highly cost-effective option.

In Birmingham, we were recently able to compare the characteristics of patients with intestinal failure referred for consideration for small bowel transplantation, according to whether or not they were referred from a unit with a multidisciplinary nutritional care team (Figure 2). Patients from nutritional care teams were significantly older at referral and each central venous catheter had lasted for significantly longer. There is therefore a strong case for developing a nutritional care team in a large centre which cares for children with intestinal failure.

Further reading

1. Beath SV, Booth IW, Kelly DA. Nutritional support in liver disease. *Archives of Disease in Childhood* 1993; **69**: 545–9
2. Rawasdeh MO, Lloyd DR, Puntis JWL, Brown GA, Booth IW. Using the steatocrit to determine optimal fat content in modular feeds. *Archives of Disease in Childhood* 1992; **67**: 608–12
3. Papadopoulou A, Rawasdeh MO, Brown GA, McNeish AS, Booth IW. Remission following an elemental diet for prednisolone in Crohn's disease. *Acta Paediatrica* (in press)
4. Beath SV, Holden C, Kelly DA, McKiernan PJ, *et al.* Role of nutritional care teams in children awaiting small bowel and liver transplantation. *Journal of Pediatric Gastroenterology and Nutrition* 1994; **19**: 337
5. Booth IW. Gastroenterology. In: McLaren DS, Burman D, Belton NR, Williams AF, eds. *Textbook of paediatric nutrition*, 3rd edn. Edinburgh: Churchill Livingstone, 1991: 143–85
6. Booth IW. Enteral nutrition in childhood. *British Journal of Hospital Medicine* 1991; **46**: 111–3
7. Puntis JWL, Booth IW. The place of a nutritional care team in paediatric practice. *Intensive Therapy and Clinical Monitoring* 1990; **11**: 132–6
8. Booth IW. Enteral nutrition as a primary therapy in short bowel syndrome. *Gut* 1994; (Suppl 1): S69–72

11 | Nutrition in cystic fibrosis

John A Dodge
Professor of Child Health, Department of Child Health,
Institute of Clinical Science, Belfast

Early descriptions of cystic fibrosis (CF) emphasised the malnutrition and associated vitamin deficiencies which were characteristic of the untreated disease. Deaths from acute respiratory infection and even bronchiectasis were commonplace among young children in the pre-antibiotic era, and children with CF would have been regarded as particularly vulnerable. With clinical recognition of the disorder, a large measure of control of the digestive problems was achieved by supplementary pancreatic enzymes, and the need for high doses of vitamins was quickly recognised. Indeed, the first clear account of CF published in 1933 was reported under the title of 'vitamin A deficiency in infants'.[1] Since those early days, management of CF in children, and more particularly in adults, has tended to drift away from clinicians with a special interest in gastrointestinal and nutritional problems to those with a major interest in respiratory disease. Now that there is general agreement on the principles of treatment for respiratory disease and on the need to apply an aggressive approach to respiratory infection, the importance of nutrition is again emerging.

Pathophysiology

Cystic fibrosis is an excellent example of a condition in which narrow 'system' specialisation is inappropriate, and the patient's social, clinical and emotional needs are recognised to be at least the apparent sum of their systematic parts. Whatever their original training, CF physicians soon find that they need to develop a wide range of knowledge and skills if they are to serve their patients adequately.

The gene responsible for CF is widely expressed throughout the body, but particularly in tissues derived from the primitive gut (which includes the lungs). Its mutations result in a variable degree of impairment of chloride movement across cell membranes, and it is believed that the gene product, cystic fibrosis transmembrane regulator (CFTR), may not be merely a chloride channel but may also have other functions, possibly as an energy-requiring pump for more complex molecules and/or a regulatory protein for cell membrane trafficking.

The precise way in which these known and putative functions in the enterocyte may affect gut absorptive mechanisms is not fully understood, but the major factor influencing fat and protein digestion and absorption ('digestibility') is whether or not the patient has pancreatic insufficiency. In the UK, only a small proportion of patients with CF retain adequate pancreatic function after the first year of life, and the precise genetic mutation (genotype) largely,[2] but not entirely,[3] determines the pancreatic status (phenotype). Pancreatic-insufficient patients, if untreated, suffer from steatorrhoea and will also rapidly become deficient in fat-soluble vitamins—though, in contrast to patients with steatorrhoea from other causes such as biliary atresia or coeliac disease, they rarely show clinical evidence of vitamin D deficiency. Characteristically, there is early marked biochemical (and sometimes clinical) evidence of deficiency of the antioxidant vitamins A and E.[4] This may indicate that excessive peroxidation of unsaturated fatty acids is part of the complex intracellular metabolic disturbance found in CF.[5]

In the age of molecular medicine and five years after the CF gene was discovered, there is still plenty of scope for the medical scientist to pursue explanations for paradoxical and puzzling clinical observations.

Energy balance

Contrary to popular belief, most CF patients left to themselves eat less than they need. There are a number of reasons for this, but depression, breathlessness and malaise are important causes of anorexia in the individual with advanced CF. Unless particular attention has been paid to maintenance of body weight, most CF patients are underweight for their height by the time they reach adulthood. There is good evidence from North America that a strong emphasis on maintaining body weight by nutritional means correlates well with improved survival. The difference in mortality between different CF clinics with similar approaches to the management of respiratory disease has been explained by differences in nutritional management.[6] Whether normal growth in childhood and the maintenance of a steady body weight in adult life can be achieved depends on maintaining in equilibrium the balance

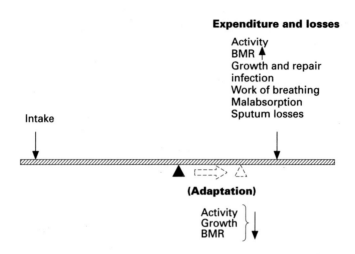

Fig. 1. *Energy balance in cystic fibrosis* (reprinted, with permission, from Ref. 7) (BMR = basal metabolic rate).

between the energy requirements of the patient and his or her energy expenditure and losses (Figure 1).[7] There is some evidence that increased energy requirements may be an intrinsic part of the basic metabolic defect,[8] at least in those who are homozygous for DF508, the commonest of the more than 500 mutations in the CF gene so far identified. A pointer to the possibility of an intrinsic heightened demand for energy was the observation that the mean birth weight of infants with CF, corrected for gestational age, is approximately 0.5 standard deviations below the population mean.[9]

The possibility of a primary increased energy requirement is still controversial, but there is general agreement that, once the stool losses have been brought under control with pancreatic enzymes, by far the most important factor determining nutritional requirements is the extent of the respiratory disease.[9,10] Interaction between nutritional state and pulmonary function is close and circular, and may be apparent even in infancy.

Clinical and biochemical evidence of malnutrition may be present within a few weeks of birth. In extreme cases, CF may present as kwashiorkor, with a florid skin rash.[11] In 9 (13%) of 66 CF infants under one year of age, low serum proteins, oedema and anaemia led to the diagnosis of protein-energy malnutrition.[12] None of these infants was taking pancreatin supplements. All five in whom it was measured had low levels of plasma zinc and, importantly, six already had their respiratory tracts colonised with *Pseudomonas aeruginosa.*

Human and animal studies have repeatedly shown that *P. aeruginosa* is particularly likely to infect malnourished individuals, yet it is common clinical experience that the first indication that a patient has become colonised with *Pseudomonas* may be a sharp fall in weight. Thus, malnutrition may predispose to pulmonary infection, while uncontrolled infection leads to weight loss. As the lung disease progresses and the work of breathing increases, so metabolic requirements increase sharply. The aim of nutritional management is to anticipate increasing needs and to develop a strategy which maintains normal growth velocity and body mass. There is abundant evidence that an aggressive approach to nutritional management may not only restore weight gain but also lead to fewer episodes of pneumonia.[13] Although good nutrition will slow the rate of deterioration in lung function, damaged lung tissue cannot be replaced except by transplantation. Established malnutrition produces a reduction in basal metabolic rate and in growth (ie adaptation).

Many biochemical parameters can be monitored but growth velocity (and particularly weight gain in childhood) remains the best clinical indicator with which to assess the adequacy or otherwise of food intake.[14] Normal growth velocity is often not achieved with energy and protein intakes below 120% of the recommended daily allowance. This need for extra food is partly explained by continuing nutrient losses in the stools, despite high intakes of pancreatin. It is usually possible to achieve at least 85% fat and protein absorption in CF patients with the use of pancreatic enzymes; in many patients, fat absorption (digestibility) of 90% or even more may be achieved.[15]

However, it must be remembered that even the most modern, high potency enzyme preparations are not perfect, and the dose-response curve is certainly not linear.[16] This means that enzyme doses may need to be doubled or even trebled to increase absorption from, say, 85% to 90%. Recent reports of colonic strictures in some young children taking very high doses have suggested that this strategy is not without risk.[17–19] (I confess to some scepticism about the need to attempt 'optimal' control of steatorrhoea in patients who are otherwise asymptomatic and growing at a normal rate.) A safe upper limit of enzyme dosage has still to be defined which, when reached, should be an indication for further investigation of the patient for a co-existing gastrointestinal disorder or for addition to the therapeutic regimen of an adjunct which improves enzyme function such as an H_2-blocker or misoprostol.

Fat is not the only nutrient lost in the stools, and there are often marked discrepancies between apparent fat and protein digestibility, as measured by balance studies.[20] It may be preferable to measure total energy lost in the stools, for which stool wet weight is a good proxy.[21]

Strategy for nutritional management

A consensus committee convened by the American Cystic Fibrosis Foundation produced guidelines in 1992 for nutritional assessment and management in CF.[22] They identified five levels of intervention, and no apology is needed for recommending their document as a state-of-the-art guide and for using their proposed categories to indicate how the CF physician and, more particularly, the dietitian need to approach the management of their patients over a period which is likely to extend over several decades (Table 1). In this schedule, it is implicit that even asymptomatic patients must be kept under frequent and regular review so that exacerbations of infection, and other complications of CF such as diabetes or liver disease, may be identified at the earliest possible opportunity and their nutritional consequences prevented or repaired.

In the first part of their report, on the assumption that patients with CF are being reviewed every 3–4 months, the consensus committee recommended that at each visit height, weight, mid-arm circumference and triceps skinfold thickness should be measured, and also head circumference in infants under the age of two years. Annual nutritional assessments should include review of dietary intake, a complete blood count and measurements of serum or plasma retinol and α-tocopherol. Other biochemical indices, including a three-day fat balance, should be measured, as indicated by clinical features such as weight loss or growth failure, as well as at the time of initial diagnosis. Armed with this information, the dietitian and clinician can tailor their nutritional recommendations accordingly.

Routine management

The dietitian is an essential member of the CF team, and her input into the care package is never more important than at the time of diagnosis. There are many valid reasons for encouraging mothers of CF patients to breast feed, perhaps the most persuasive being its

Table 1. Categories for nutritional management of patients with cystic fibrosis (CF) (reprinted, with permission, from Ref. 22)

Category	Target group	Goals
Routine management	All CF patients	Nutritional education, dietary counselling, pancreatic-enzyme replacement (for patients with PI), vitamin supplementation (for patients with PI).
Anticipatory guidance	CF patients at risk of developing energy imbalance (ie severe PI, frequent pulmonary infections, periods of rapid growth), but maintaining a weight-height index ≥90% of ideal weight.	Further education to prepare patients for increased energy needs; increased monitoring of dietary intake; increase caloric density in diet as needed; behavioural assessment and counselling.
Supportive intervention	Patients with decreased weight velocity and/or a weight-height index 85–90% of ideal weight.	All of the above plus oral supplements as needed.
Rehabilitative care	Patients with a weight-height index consistently <85% of ideal weight.	All of the above plus enteral supplementation via nasogastric tube or enterostomy as indicated.
Resuscitative and palliative care	Patients with a weight-height index <75% of ideal weight, or progressive nutritional failure.	All of the above plus continuous enteral feeds or total parenteral nutrition.

value to the mother in boosting her confidence and reducing the (inappropriate) guilt feelings that so many mothers experience when coming to terms with the inherited nature of CF—but there are also some theoretical and practical problems. The relatively low protein content of breast milk compared with cow's milk formula is, in this instance, a potential disadvantage. It is no coincidence that the occasional cases of protein-energy malnutrition in undiagnosed CF patients occur predominantly among breast fed or soy milk fed babies. Most CF centres advise breast feeding mothers to continue, but the great majority of CF infants have pancreatic insufficiency and will require pancreatic enzyme supplements which must be given separately during the course of a feed. For others, a standard infant formula (with enzymes) or a hydrolysed formula (with enzymes when solids are introduced) is recommended. The infant who has had extensive resection for meconium ileus presents a special problem, and will often require nasogastric feeding.

It has already been stated that early vitamin A and E deficiencies occur in the untreated patient. In a recent review[23] it was recommended that vitamins A and D should be given in double the standard dosage for age, and that all patients should also take vitamin E, 30–200 mg/day according to age, in liquid or tablet form. Patients with liver disease may also require vitamin K. There may be an additional requirement for carotenoids other than β-carotene. Carotenoids are potent antioxidants with the ability to quench oxygen free radicals;[24] there is a negative correlation between carotenoid levels and indices of inflammation, but no correlation with fat absorption. No vitamin product currently available in the UK meets all requirements, although one which has been developed specifically for CF patients in the USA may soon become available here.

Anticipatory guidance

Oral intake needs to be boosted during and after pulmonary infection and periods of rapid growth. This can usually be achieved by increasing the energy density of the normal diet, mainly by adding fat and, of course, by increasing pancreatic enzymes appropriately. Energy-rich supplements can usually be prepared using normal foods, and families not infrequently find themselves in the paradoxical situation in which the CF child is encouraged to eat large amounts of energy-rich 'junk' foods which their parents and healthy siblings are exhorted to avoid. The importance of regular contact with the dietitian for education and supervision is obvious, and at times the help of a psychologist can be invaluable in devising a suitable behavioural programme.[25]

Supportive intervention

When children with CF fail to maintain their weight velocity or actually lose weight, there is a need for early and aggressive nutritional intervention. Energy-rich drinks initially supplement (but do not replace) the child's normal diet, and experience shows that supplements based on milk are likely to be as effective as the more expensive predigested or elemental products. When the volume required exceeds the patient's willingness or ability to take, enteral feeds need to be given by nasogastric tube or gastrostomy. Nasogastric tubes may be useful in the short term but gastrostomy is much better tolerated.

The decision to place a gastrostomy marks a major milestone in the progress of the disease and needs to be fully discussed with the patient and the family. In patients with impaired glucose tolerance, who comprise a significant proportion of adolescents and young adults, enteral feeding may produce frank diabetes mellitus. Gastrooesophageal reflux, which is common in CF, may also be unmasked or precipitated by gastrostomy feeds. Care givers need to be aware of and alert for these possibilities, so that appropriate action can be taken.

There is a growing literature on the short- and long-term benefits of enteral nutrition in CF, and it would be fair to say that there is still incomplete agreement about its long-term value. It may have a particular place in maintaining body weight in CF patients with advanced lung disease who are on the waiting list for lung transplantation. Parenteral nutrition, on the other hand, is nearly always suitable only for short-term support and rehabilitation. It may have a particular value in young infants after intestinal resection for meconium ileus, or for those few older patients in whom resection has become necessary for intussusception or other intestinal problems.

Conclusions

A wide range of techniques and products is available for support and rehabilitation of patients with nutritional deficiency. Nevertheless, the objectives of treatment should be to anticipate and prevent the onset of nutritional problems, or at least to postpone them for as long as possible. This is best achieved by a policy of frequent and careful surveillance, in which an experienced dietitian plays a major role.

References

1. Blackfan KD, Wolbach SB. Vitamin A deficiency in infants. *Journal of Pediatrics* 1933; **6**: 679–706
2. Kerem E, Corey M, Kerem B-S, Rommens J, *et al.* The relation between genotype and phenotype in cystic fibrosis—analysis of the most common mutation. *New England Journal of Medicine* 1990; **323**: 1517–22

3. The Cystic Fibrosis Genotype-Phenotype Consortium. Correlation between genotype and phenotype in patients with cystic fibrosis. *New England Journal of Medicine* 1993; **329**: 1308–13

4. Sokol RJ, Reardon MC, Accurso FJ, Stool C, *et al.* Fat-soluble vitamin status during the first year of life in infants with cystic fibrosis identified by screening of newborns. *American Journal of Clinical Nutrition* 1989; **50**: 1064–71

5. Salh B, Webb K, Guyan PM, Day JP, *et al.* Aberrant free radical activity in cystic fibrosis. *Clinica Chimica Acta* 1989; **181**: 65–74

6. Corey M, McLaughlin FJ, Williams M, Levison H. A comparison of survival, growth, and pulmonary function in patients with cystic fibrosis in Boston and Toronto. *Journal of Clinical Epidemiology* 1988; **41**: 583–91

7. Dodge JA, O'Rawe AM. Energy requirements in cystic fibrosis. In: Dodge JA, Brock DJH, Widdicombe JH, eds. *Cystic fibrosis—current topics*, Vol. 12. Chichester: John Wiley & Sons, 1994: 233–52

8. O'Rawe A, McIntosh I, Dodge JA, Brock DJH, *et al.* Increased energy expenditure in cystic fibrosis is associated with specific mutations. *Clinical Science* 1992; **82**: 71–6

9. Hsia DY. Birth weight in cystic fibrosis of the pancreas. *Annals of Human Genetics* 1959; **23**: 289–99

10. Pencharz PB, Durie PR. Nutritional management of cystic fibrosis. *Annual Reviews of Nutrition* 1993; **13**: 111–36

11. Phillips RJ, Crock CN, Dillon MJ, Clayton PT, *et al.* Cystic fibrosis presenting as kwashiorkor with florid skin rash. *Archives of Disease in Childhood* 1993; **69**: 446–8

12. Abman SH, Accurso FJ, Bowman CM. Persistent morbidity and mortality of protein calorie malnutrition in young infants with cystic fibrosis. *Journal of Pediatric Gastroenterology and Nutrition* 1986; **5**: 393–6

13. O'Loughlin EV, Forbes D, Parsons H, Scott B, *et al.* Nutritional rehabilitation in malnourished children with cystic fibrosis: effect on the course of the disease. In: Lawson D, ed. *Cystic fibrosis horizons.* Chichester: John Wiley & Sons, 1984: 97

14. Dodge JA. Nutrition in cystic fibrosis: a historical overview. *Proceedings of the Nutrition Society* 1992; **51**: 225–35

15. Beker LT, Fink RJ, Shamsa FH, Chaney HR, *et al.* Comparison of weight-based dosages of enteric-coated microtablet enzyme preparations in patients with cystic fibrosis. *Journal of Pediatric Gastroenterology and Nutrition* 1994; **19**: 191–7

16. Lebenthal E, Rolston DDK, Holsclaw DS. Enzyme therapy for pancreatic insufficiency: present status and future needs. *Pancreas* 1994; **1**: 1–12

17. Smyth RL, van Velzen D, Smyth AR, Lloyd DA, Heaf DP. Strictures of ascending colon in cystic fibrosis and high-strength pancreatic enzymes. *Lancet* 1994; **343**: 85–6

18. Oades DJ, Bush A, Ong PS, Brereton RJ. High-strength pancreatic enzyme supplements and large bowel stricture in cystic fibrosis [letter]. *Lancet* 1994; **343**: 109

19. Taylor CJ. Colonic strictures in cystic fibrosis. *Lancet* 1994; **343**: 615–6

20. Morrison JM, O'Rawe A, McCracken KJ, Redmond AOB, Dodge JA. Energy intakes and losses in cystic fibrosis. *Journal of Human Nutrition and Dietetics* 1994; **7**: 39–46

21. Murphy JL, Wootton SA, Bond SA, Jackson AA. Energy content of stools in normal healthy controls and patients with cystic fibrosis. *Archives of Disease in Childhood* 1991; **66**: 495–500

22. Ramsey BW, Farrell PM, Pencharz P and the Consensus Committee. Nutritional assessment and management in cystic fibrosis: a consensus report. *American Journal of Clinical Nutrition* 1992; **55**: 108–16

23. Peters SA, Rolles CJ. Vitamin therapy in cystic fibrosis—a review and rationale. *Journal of Clinical Pharmacology and Therapeutics* 1993; **18**: 33–8

24. Homnick DN, Cow JH, DeLoof MJ, Ringer TV. Carotenoid levels in normal children and in children with cystic fibrosis. *Journal of Pediatrics* 1993; **122**; 703–7

25. Stark LJ, Bowen AM, Tyc VL, Evans S, Passero MA. A behavioural approach to increasing calorie consumption in children with cystic fibrosis. *Journal of Paediatric Psychology* 1990; **15**: 309–26

12 | Nutrition in renal disease

Alan R Watson
Consultant Paediatric Nephrologist and Director, Paediatric Renal Unit,
City Hospital, Nottingham

Nutrition is an important aspect of the management of children with renal disorders. Such children may have fluctuating clinical and biochemical disturbances, and nutritional goals require frequent readjustment with advice from an experienced dietitian. Children with complicated nephrotic syndrome and acute and chronic renal failure will usually be treated in a designated paediatric renal unit where nutritional advice is one aspect of support from the multidisciplinary team.

This chapter will cover some aspects of nutrition in renal disorders. Readers are referred to other texts for further dietetic and clinical details.[1-3]

Nephrotic syndrome

The majority of children with nephrotic syndrome have a steroid-responsive lesion with normal renal function, and it is assumed that they have minimal histological change in the glomeruli (MCNS: minimal change nephrotic syndrome). The main clinical problems occur during their first admission to hospital with oedema. During this phase, fluid restriction and diuretics may be necessary as it may take 1–3 weeks before corticosteroids induce a remission with diuresis and loss of protein in the urine.[4]

Early work suggested that high protein diets promote increased albumin synthesis, but such diets have little effect on serum albumin concentrations. The current recommendation is to promote a healthy eating diet for all the family, with an adequate energy intake based on the estimated average requirement for children of the same chronological age.[5] A protein intake of 1–2 g/kg body weight/day should be adequate for most children. During the oedematous phase it is particularly important to stress a 'no added salt' diet; this should be followed as part of the long-term general healthy eating advice. A very low sodium diet and the use of low sodium specialist products are not necessary.

Hyperlipidaemia

Grossly elevated cholesterol and triglyceride levels are part of the nephrotic syndrome. The use of mono- or poly-unsaturated margarines and oils is included in the general healthy eating advice together with the reduction of saturated fat intake. Drug therapy to lower lipid levels is not necessary in children with steroid-responsive nephrotic syndrome, but it is a current issue in those who are steroid-resistant and have persistently elevated serum lipids.[6] We have shown in a recent study (Coleman JE, Watson AR. Submitted for publication) that dietary therapy alone in such children lowered cholesterol and triglycerides by 8% and 14%, respectively. However, the addition of the hydroxymethylglutaryl-CoA reductase inhibitor simvastatin lowered cholesterol levels to within the normal range in the majority of patients within a few months (mean reduction, 41%), with triglyceride levels also significantly reduced (44% reduction).

Food allergy

Some reports suggest that food hypersensitivity, particularly to milk and dairy products, may play a part in relapses in children with nephrotic syndrome.[7] The aetiology of MCNS is unclear, so some parents may be concerned that dietary factors might be responsible. Paediatricians need to be aware of this as some children have been referred for homoeopathic therapy. If a trial of a few-foods diet is contemplated, it should be under close dietetic supervision.

Steroid-dependent nephrotic syndrome

Children who require frequent or continuous steroid therapy may experience side-effects of obesity, muscle wasting, osteopenia and growth retardation.[8] Hopefully, many of these complications can be avoided using prolonged courses of alternate-day prednisolone or other immunosuppressive drugs. Frequent dietetic review and support may be necessary to restrict excessive energy intake, again reinforced by healthy eating advice.

Steroid-resistant nephrotic syndrome

The rare child with congenital nephrotic syndrome or the 'malignant' type of focal segmental glomerular sclerosis (FSGS) may have severe protein malnutrition underlying the grossly oedematous state. Energy intake should be maximised within the fluid allowance together with a protein intake of 3–4 g/kg body weight/day. Children with conditions such as FSGS often progress to end-stage renal failure. Children with congenital nephrotic syndrome often have normal renal function, but their previously invariably fatal prognosis has now been replaced through a policy of aggressive management with nasogastric or gastrostomy feeding, combined with bilateral nephrectomy and commencement of dialysis with renal transplantation in mind.[9]

Acute renal failure

Acute renal failure (ARF) is characterised by a sudden decrease in renal function with retention of nitrogenous wastes and disturbance of water and electrolyte homoeostasis. Most children are oliguric, but some have marked polyuria, especially after relief of urinary obstruction such as might occur after ablation of posterior urethral valves.[10] Haemolytic uraemic syndrome is now the commonest cause of ARF in childhood in the UK and typically follows a prodromal illness of diarrhoea which is often bloody. Patients with ARF are often catabolic, particularly if the problem is acute tubular necrosis in association with sepsis, burns and/or trauma.

Some children who are not highly catabolic may be conservatively managed without dialysis. However, in this situation fluid intake needs to be restricted to the previous day's output plus insensible losses, and often there is little fluid allowance in which to deliver the nutritional prescription. Dialysis is often undertaken at an early stage with the benefit of creating 'nutritional space'. Peritoneal dialysis is usually favoured, but haemodialysis and haemofiltration techniques may be required.

Nutritional management of acute renal failure
Adequate nutrition in ARF will help to:

- ameliorate catabolism and reduce the rate of solute production;
- maintain a good nutritional state and possibly improve resistance to infection; and
- hasten recovery and renal healing.

The dietary principles are an energy supplemented, reduced

Table 1. Guidelines for energy and protein intakes in acute renal failure.

	*Energy (kcal/kg body wt/day)	Protein (g/kg body wt/day)
Conservative management		
0–2 yr	95–150	1.0–1.8
Children/adolescents	minimum of EAR for height age	1.0
Peritoneal dialysis		
0–2 yr	95–150	**2.0–2.5
Children/adolescents	minimum of EAR for height age	1.0–2.5
Haemodialysis		
0–2 yr	95–150	1.5–2.1
Children/adolescents	minimum of EAR for height age	1.0–1.8

*Guidelines, rarely achieved in the acute stage because of fluid restriction.
**If dialysis is prolonged, increased protein may be required.
EAR = estimated average requirement (Dietary reference values, 1991).[12]

protein diet with appropriate potassium, sodium and phosphate restriction.[11] Guidelines for energy and protein intakes are shown in Table 1.

Methods of feeding

Some children with ARF may initially take oral fluids because of thirst, but most of them fail to meet the necessary nutritional goals via the oral route. A comparison of oral versus nasogastric feeding in children with haemolytic uraemic syndrome was attempted in our unit, but the study was soon abandoned as it became clear that nasogastric feeding more effectively achieved nutritional goals. If children need sedation for the insertion of dialysis catheters and/or arterial lines, a fine bore nasogastric tube is routinely placed.[10] Continuous 24-hour tube feeding using an enteral feeding pump may be advantageous in the initial stages of treatment, with transition to overnight feeding as oral intake improves and the child recovers.

Total parenteral nutrition. This route is considered only if enteral nutrition is not tolerated. A total parenteral nutrition regimen has to be modified for the child with ARF because of fluid restriction and electrolyte composition. Medical staff need to liaise closely with the dietitian as daily prescription may change depending upon electrolyte and fluid balance status. The use of high nitrogen, electrolyte-free solutions can be considered (eg Vamin 18EF or 14EF) to provide increased energy from carbohydrate and fat solutions (50% dextrose, Intralipid 20%) if fluid intake is limited.

Chronic renal failure

Children with chronic renal failure (CRF) provide the major workload for specialist paediatric renal units where the disadvantages of travel are offset by benefits of access to a multidisciplinary team and the essential input of an experienced dietitian. In the past, many children with CRF suffered marked growth retardation and, as a result, a more aggressive approach to nutritional management has now been adopted.[13]

CRF may be described as:

- mild (50–80 ml/min/1.73 m^2);
- moderate (20–50 ml/min/1.73 m^2); or
- severe (10–20 ml/min/1.73 m^2).

Biochemical abnormalities and some non-specific symptoms may develop during moderate CRF. As the condition advances, ill health and growth failure become apparent. Dialysis in children is seen only as a holding measure before renal transplantation is carried out, with an increasing trend to transplant children before dialysis is required (pre-emptive transplantation).

Conservative management

During the pre-dialysis stage, the nutritional aims are to:

- maintain normal growth;
- prevent uraemic symptoms (eg nausea and vomiting);
- slow progression to end-stage renal failure that requires dialysis and transplantation; and
- attempt to maintain 'normal' family routines with nursery and school attendance.

Regular assessment of the child in the clinic with accurate growth monitoring is essential if growth faltering is to be detected early and other modifications to the diet or dialysis implemented. Frequent biochemical assessment, combined with information from growth parameters, dietetic interview and three-day food diaries, are used to construct an overall treatment plan for each child.

In recent years there has been much interest in low protein diets to slow the progression of CRF. However, after an initial enthusiasm, they have not been universally adopted, especially in children in whom there are concerns about causing malnutrition and growth failure as well as problems with practical implementation.[14]

Nutritional guidelines for the child with CRF are shown in Table 2. The provision of adequate energy is essential to promote growth, particularly during the pre-dialysis stage of treatment. Although high energy, low protein foods are encouraged, in practice energy supplements are usually relied upon to achieve the child's requirements.

Energy supplements. Combined fat and carbohydrate supplements (eg Duocal powder) can be successfully added to infant formula. Liquid glucose polymers are more popular if diluted with a fizzy drink or squash, but the volume permitted will depend on fluid allowance. Powdered glucose polymers are useful for those children who drink plenty of water, squash or baby juice. The use of measured volumes and scoops ensures better compliance at home.

Protein requirements are generally reduced during conservative management to minimise uraemia and control hyperphosphataemia. Protein-containing supplements are rarely required prior to dialysis as most children usually receive sufficient protein from infant formula and/or diet.

The protein requirements of children on chronic peritoneal dialysis can be generally increased to allow for the reported dialysis losses of protein and albumin. However, cow's milk and other dairy products must be restricted if hyperphosphataemia is to be controlled. Protein intake of children undergoing haemodialysis should be regulated to minimise fluctuations in pre-dialysis blood urea levels. Protein exchange lists are of limited use as the majority of children do not take kindly to low protein foods which are on prescription.

Fluid and electrolytes. Each child's requirements will need assessing individually because some children with dysplastic kidneys are salt losers who require additional sodium supplements. Other children have particular problems with salt and water retention. Hyperkalaemia may be a major problem in children on haemodialysis, particularly those with poor native renal function.

Renal osteodystrophy. The prevention and treatment of renal osteodystrophy has been transformed by the availability of vitamin D

Table 2. Guidelines for energy and protein intakes in chronic renal failure.

	Energy (kcal/kg body wt/day)	Protein (g/kg body wt/day)
Pre-dialysis		
Infants		
Pre-term	120–180	2.5–3.0
0–0.5 yr	115–150	1.5–2.1
0.5–1.0 yr	95–150	1.5–1.8
1.0–2.0 yr	95–120	1.0–1.8
Children/adolescents		
2.0–puberty	minimum of EAR	1.0–1.5
pubertal	for height age	1.0–1.5
post-pubertal		1.0–1.5
Peritoneal dialysis (CAPD/CCPD)		
Infants		
Pre-term	120–180	3.0–4.0
0–0.5 yr	115–150	2.1–3.0
0.5–1.0 yr	95–150	2.0–3.0
1.0–2.0 yr	95–120	2.0–3.0
Children/adolescents		
2.0–puberty	minimum of EAR	2.5
pubertal	for height age	2.0
post-pubertal		1.5
Haemodialysis		
Infants		
Pre-term	120–180	3.0
0–0.5 yr	115–150	2.1
0.5–1.0 yr	95–150	1.5–2.0
1.0–2.0 yr	95–120	1.5–1.8
Children/adolescents		
2.0–puberty	minimum of EAR	1.0–1.5
pubertal	for height age	1.0–1.5
post-pubertal		1.0–1.5

CAPD = continuous ambulatory peritoneal dialysis.
CCPD = chronic cycling peritoneal dialysis.
EAR = estimated average requirement (Dietary reference values, 1991).[12]

analogues which can substitute for the hormone 1,25-dihydroxy-cholecalciferol which is normally formed in the proximal renal tubule.[15,16] Maintaining a normal serum calcium and phosphate biochemistry is crucial for normal bone growth, and nutritional measures have a large part to play here. In moderate and severe CRF the great reduction in the amount of inorganic phosphate filtered by the glomeruli leads to a rise in plasma phosphate and a fall in ionised calcium which stimulates parathyroid hormone release. Reducing dietary phosphate intake is therefore an essential step in preventing or reversing hyperparathyroidism. Alkali therapy to control the chronic metabolic acidosis may be of equal importance.

Traditional infant formulas are low in phosphate, and any nutritional supplements should contain as little phosphate as possible and be included within the dietary allowance. As general guidelines, phosphate should be restricted to:

- 200–300 mg/day in infants;
- 400–600 mg/day in children <20 kg body weight; and
- 600–800 mg/day in children >20 kg body weight.

Phosphate binders. Calcium carbonate is now the first choice phosphate binder (aluminium hydroxide has largely been abandoned because of potential aluminium deposition in bone and brain). Compliance is always a major problem, and the choice of a suitable powder or tablet might require discussion with the child and family.

Micronutrients. Little is known about the micronutrient requirements of infants and children with CRF. Children most at risk of micronutrient deficiencies are those:

- anorexic with vomiting and not receiving nutritional support;
- remaining on restricted diets for prolonged periods of time (ie conservatively managed);
- undergoing prolonged dialysis while awaiting transplantation;
- with episodes of peritonitis; and/or
- receiving erythropoietin.

Ketovite tablets, 2–3 a day, will ensure intake of vitamins C, E and the B complex and are generally well tolerated. Ketovite liquid and Abidec should be avoided because of their vitamin A content. A recent survey of UK units suggested that a great variety of micronutrient supplements are currently in use within the UK and

Ireland; further work is required to assess the need for comprehensive and palatable supplements.[17]

Nutritional support methods. Whenever possible, nutritional supplements are encouraged by the oral route, but experience has shown that attempting to achieve an adequate oral intake can be difficult and stressful for the parents. It is now more common for supplementary feeds to be given by the nasogastric or gastrostomy route. Nasogastric tubes are popular in many units, but have the disadvantage of needing frequent replacement; gastrostomy feeding using a gastrostomy button device is in the long term far more aesthetically pleasing.[18,19]

Vomiting can be a persistent problem, especially in infants, and the feeding prescription should be monitored and altered appropriately. The families of these children require a great deal of support by members of the multidisciplinary team. Many are heard to remark that the dialysis is easy—it is the feeding that is difficult.

Renal transplantation

One of the undoubted benefits of renal transplantation is the increase in appetite, and energy intake may often have to be restricted to avoid the initial rapid weight gain on high-dose corticosteroids. A healthy eating diet is encouraged.

Conclusions

Nutritional advice is essential in the management of children with renal disorders. Constant adjustments are needed to promote growth while taking into account the biochemical and treatment changes. The involvement of an experienced dietitian is mandatory, and all members of the multidisciplinary team have a role to play in maintaining good nutrition in these children.

References

1. Coleman JE. The kidney. In: Shaw V, Lawson M, eds. *Clinical paediatric dietetics.* London: Blackwell Scientific Publications, 1994: 125–42
2. Haycock GB. Renal disease. In: McLaren DS, Burman D, Belton NR, Williams AF, eds. *Textbook of paediatric nutrition*, 3rd edn. Edinburgh: Churchill Livingstone, 1991: 237–56
3. Weiss RA. Dietary and pharmacologic treatment of chronic renal failure. In: Edelman CM Jr, ed. *Pediatric kidney disease*, 2nd edn. Boston, MA: Little Brown, 1992: 815–25

4. British Association for Paediatric Nephrology, and Research Unit Royal College of Physicians. Consensus statement on management and audit potential for steroid responsive nephrotic syndrome. Report of a workshop. *Archives of Disease in Childhood* 1994; **70**: 151–7

5. Watson AR, Coleman JE. Dietary management in nephrotic syndrome. *Archives of Disease in Childhood* 1993; **69**: 179–80

6. Thomas ME, Harris KPG, Ramaswamy C, Hattersley JM, *et al.* Simvastatin therapy for hypercholesterolemic patients with nephrotic syndrome or significant proteinuria. *Kidney International* 1993; **44**: 1124–9

7. Lagrue G, Laurent J, Rostoker G, Lang P. Food allergy in idiopathic nephrotic syndrome [letter]. *Lancet* 1987; **ii**: 277

8. Rees L, Greene SA, Adlard P, Jones J, *et al.* Growth and endocrine function in steroid sensitive nephrotic syndrome. *Archives of Disease in Childhood* 1988; **63**: 484–90

9. Rapola J, Huttunen NP, Hallman N. Congenital and infantile nephrotic syndrome. In: Edelman CM Jr, ed. *Pediatric kidney disease*, 2nd edn. Boston, MA: Little Brown, 1992: 1291–305

10. Watson AR. The management of acute renal failure. *Current Paediatrics* 1991; **1**: 103–7

11. Coleman JE, Watson AR. Nutritional support for the child with acute renal failure. *Journal of Human Nutrition and Dietetics* 1992; **5**: 99–105

12. Department of Health. *Dietary reference values for food and energy nutrients for the United Kingdom.* Reports on Health and Social Subjects, No. 41. London: HMSO, 1991

13. Rees L, Rigden SPA, Ward GM. Chronic renal failure and growth. *Archives of Disease in Childhood* 1989; **64**: 573–7

14. Raymond NG, Dwyer JT, Nevins P, Kurtin P. An approach to protein restriction in children with renal insufficiency. *Pediatric Nephrology* 1990; **4**: 145–51

15. Watson AR, Kooh SW, Tam CS, Reilly BJ, *et al.* Renal osteodystrophy in children on CAPD: a prospective trial of 1-alpha-hydroxycholecalciferol therapy. *Child Nephrology and Urology* 1988; **9**: 220–7

16. Salusky IB, Ramirez J, Goodman WG. Disorders of bone and mineral metabolism in chronic renal failure. In: Holliday MA, Barratt TM, Avner ED, eds. *Pediatric nephrology*, 3rd edn. Baltimore, MD: Williams & Wilkins, 1993: 1287–304

17. Coleman JE, Fyfe A, Watson AR. Micronutrient supplements for chronic renal failure: a survey of paediatric practice. *Journal of Renal Nutrition* (in press)

18. Conley SB. Supplemental (NG) feedings of infants undergoing continuous peritoneal dialysis. In: Fine RN, ed. *Chronic ambulatory peritoneal dialysis (CAPD) and chronic cycling peritoneal dialysis (CCPD) in children.* Boston, MA: Nijhoff, 1987: 263–9

19. Coleman JE, Watson AR. Gastrostomy buttons: the optimal route for nutritional support in children with chronic renal failure. *Journal of Renal Nutrition* 1992; **2**: 21–6

13 Feeding and nutrition in children with cerebral palsy

Jonathan M Couriel
Consultant in Paediatrics and Paediatric Respiratory Medicine,
Booth Hall Children's Hospital, Manchester School of Medicine

> Joseph moved locked, lost limbs in involuntary movements. Joseph always carped, always appealing for time to tackle tame and timid efforts to eat. Eating, poor Joseph found, took toll of everyone's patience.[1]
>
> (Christopher Nolan, aged 11,
> athetoid cerebral palsy sufferer)

For most children, eating is a source of happiness. Mealtimes are an intimate aspect of family life which play an important role in a child's social development, but for many children with cerebral palsy and other neurodevelopmental handicaps, and for their parents, each meal is a distressing and time-consuming necessity rather than a pleasure.[1–5] Meals are punctuated by repeated spillage, coughing, choking and regurgitation. The child may feel frightened, frustrated, uncomfortable or embarrassed. Many parents find meals stressful, whilst others feel guilty because they cannot achieve an adequate intake of food. Feeding difficulties are often the major hurdle in the parents' day-to-day care of their handicapped child.

What are the causes and effects of feeding problems in these children, and how can these problems best be assessed and managed?

Prevalence of feeding difficulties in cerebral palsy

Cerebral palsy is the commonest cause of neurological handicap in children, affecting approximately two in every 1,000, or a total of 200,000 children in the UK. Eating difficulties are common in children with cerebral palsy; as would be expected, the more severe the degree of handicap, the more severe the feeding problems. Overall, 40–60% of children with cerebral palsy have some difficulty with eating, but 85% of those with spastic quadriplegia have severe difficulties,[6] and 50–60% of young disabled adults have feeding problems. In a recent population-based study of 50 pre-school children with cerebral palsy, 90% had significant and 36% severe oromotor dysfunction.[7]

Aetiology of feeding problems in cerebral palsy

Many factors contribute to the eating difficulties experienced by these children. Abnormal or poorly coordinated movements of the mouth, pharynx and oesophagus are often the most important. This is not surprising since safe, efficient swallowing requires the coordination of six cranial nerves, the brain-stem and cerebral cortex, and 26 muscles of the mouth, pharynx and oesophagus.[8–10] Abnormal body posture, poor head control and, in some children, involuntary movements or frequent seizures compound the problem. Impaired hearing or vision and poor comprehension make communication difficult. As previous experiences of feeding have often been traumatic, some children develop aversive patterns of behaviour when their mouth or face is touched.

Normal and abnormal swallowing

Normal swallowing consists of two voluntary phases (oral preparatory and oral) followed by two reflex phases (pharyngeal and oesophageal). Each phase depends on the phase preceding it, but this complex sequence is disrupted in the handicapped child:

- In the *oral preparatory phase*, food is formed into a bolus. This requires sealing of the lips, chewing, and the cupping of the bolus in a depression in the tongue. Abnormal oral sensation, involuntary movements or behavioural problems can interfere with this phase.

- In the *oral phase*, the tongue propels the bolus backwards. Many children with cerebral palsy have tongue thrust, in which the tongue moves anteriorly before moving posteriorly.

- When the bolus passes the anterior fauces and enters the pharynx, the swallowing reflex is triggered; from this point, the process is involuntary. In this *pharyngeal phase*, the soft palate rises against the posterior pharynx to prevent nasal regurgitation. The bolus is propelled by peristalsis of the pharyngeal constrictors to the cricopharyngeal sphincter of the oesophagus. Simultaneously, the larynx moves upwards and forwards and is closed. This enlarges the pharynx and opens the oesophagus by relaxing the cricopharyngeal sphincter.

- In the *oesophageal phase*, the bolus then passes down the oesophagus by peristalsis, the lower oesophageal sphincter relaxes, and the bolus passes into the stomach.

Initiation of the swallowing reflex is often delayed or absent in children with cerebral palsy, leaving the airway inadequately protected. If the reflex is not triggered, food can accumulate in the vallecula or pyriform sinuses and then be aspirated. Poor oesophageal peristalsis and gastro-oesophageal reflux (GOR) occur in 75% of children with cerebral palsy and feeding difficulties.

Assessment of feeding in the child with neurological handicap

Three fundamental issues need to be addressed when assessing feeding in a child with cerebral palsy or other severe neurological disorder:

1. Is feeding achieving adequate nutrition?
2. Is feeding safe?
3. Is feeding efficient, comfortable and enjoyable?

Is feeding achieving adequate nutrition?

There is evidence of inadequate nutrition and poor growth in 48–94% of children with cerebral palsy.[2,3,6,11] In different studies, height, weight, weight-for-height, skinfold thickness and fat-free mass have been shown to be reduced. Feeding problems and inadequate nutrition occur more frequently in children with spastic quadriplegia than in those with a hemiplegia or diplegia.[6,12]

In a detailed study of 142 children and adolescents with spastic quadriplegia, the relationship between the severity of cognitive, ambulatory and oromotor disabilities and growth and nutritional status was assessed.[6] Growth was measured using a combination of weight, upper arm and lower leg length, skinfold thickness and pubertal staging. Median weight and triceps skinfold thickness fat stores were reduced to 65% of the median predicted normal values. Muscle stores were less affected, being 88% of the median. There was a clear correlation between the severity of oromotor dysfunction and the degree of linear growth failure: the more severe the neurological handicap, the more severe both the feeding problems and the growth failure.[6]

Malnutrition has important consequences for these children. As discussed in other chapters of this book, inadequate nutrition, particularly in early life, can lead to irreversible impairment of somatic growth and, by impairing brain growth, can add further to the developmental delay from which so many of these children already suffer. By impairing immune function, malnutrition increases the risk of serious infection. Reduced muscle strength and mobility, decreased levels of activity, motivation and attention span are all associated with inadequate nutritional intake.

Two important issues need to be considered in assessing the relationship between feeding and growth in children with cerebral palsy:

1. *How should growth and nutritional status be measured in these children?* Conventional indices such as height, weight-for-height or height velocity are often impossible to measure, for example, in the wheel-chair-bound child with kyphoscoliosis. Measurements of upper arm and lower leg length may be more helpful and reproducible in assessing linear growth.[5,13] Measurements of skinfold thickness and arm circumference are also difficult to interpret in children with cerebral palsy—they have reduced muscle and fat mass even if there are no feeding difficulties. Analysis of body composition, such as by bioelectrical impedance, may prove to be informative but is not commonly used.

There is, in fact, no agreed method of estimating the energy needs of these children. Accounting for body mass, tone and activity may be more accurate than using standard recommendations.[14]

2. *Factors other than nutrition affect growth in children with cerebral palsy.*[11,15] The child's genetic potential or a history of intra-uterine growth retardation will influence its growth. Abnormalities of the central nervous system can affect somatic growth directly. There is also controversy about whether endocrine factors such as growth hormone deficiency contribute to poor growth in these children.

Although these other factors may be important, there is no doubt that malnutrition is an important, and potentially reversible, cause of growth failure in many children with cerebral palsy. Several studies have shown that gastrostomy or nasogastric feeding of these children with energy- and protein-rich foods results in a rapid correction of wasting, an increase in weight/height ratio and an improvement in their general well-being.[16,17]

Is feeding safe?

Safe, efficient eating requires coordination of swallowing and breathing. The child with impaired swallowing has a poorly pro-tected airway and is at high risk of aspiration.[18] Recurrent respiratory symptoms are common in children with neurodevelopmental handicap and feeding problems.[3,5,19,20] Symptoms range in severity from occasional coughing with drinks to repeated episodes of pneumonia, bronchiectasis and respiratory failure. In a series of 93 children referred to the Booth Hall Children's Hospital with feeding difficulties and neurodevelopmental handicap, 44% had symptoms of significant recurrent respiratory illness.

Respiratory disease is the commonest cause of death in children with cerebral palsy.[21] In a large regional study of deaths in children and young adults with cerebral palsy, a respiratory disorder was mentioned on 78% of the death certificates.[22]

Aspiration of feeds. Aspiration that occurs at the beginning of a feed *before* swallowing has occurred suggests poor tongue control or an abnormal swallow reflex. Aspiration *during* swallowing indicates failure of laryngeal closure. Aspiration can also *follow* swallowing, with inhalation of residual food from the pharynx, or be secondary to GOR.[18]

Aspiration is the commonest cause of respiratory symptoms in this group of children, but other factors such as immobility, weak respiratory muscles, spinal and chest wall deformities, and poor cough predispose them to respiratory illness. Their immune response to infection is blunted by malnutrition. Parental smoking will increase the frequency and severity of respiratory symptoms, and a personal or family history of atopic disease in the child with wheeze and cough may suggest co-existing asthma.

Inhalation of food into the respiratory tract produces a spectrum of pathological and clinical responses.[19,20] Aspiration of milk produces acute inflammation in the airways and alveoli. The child coughs and becomes distressed, and there may be recurrent wheezing, stridor or rattly breathing. In the young infant, aspiration can cause life-threatening apnoea. If aspiration recurs over months or years, it can lead to progressive interstitial fibrosis, obliterative bronchiolitis and persistent atelectasis. Secondary infection can result in recurrent pneumonia, lung abscess formation and, in some children, bronchiectasis with a chronic productive cough.

To assess whether or not feeding is safe, a detailed history is vital. Coughing, choking, respiratory distress, stridor or wheeze during or after feeds suggests aspiration. The diagnosis of aspiration is delayed in many children with feeding problems because it can occur without any of these symptoms—some children with recurrent aspiration have a blunted or absent cough reflex. The history alone is therefore not reliable at identifying aspiration, and a radiological examination such as videofluoroscopy of swallowing is needed to detect this 'silent aspiration'. In addition to aspiration 'from the top end' during feeding, chest symptoms can follow aspiration secondary to the GOR from which so many of these children suffer.

Is feeding efficient, comfortable and enjoyable?
Asking the parents of many children with cerebral palsy to describe a typical meal demonstrates that feeding is emphatically not efficient, comfortable or enjoyable. Observing feeding in the home or clinic, either directly or with video recordings, is helpful in assessing objectively the difficulties with which both the children and the parents have to cope. For example, many parents say that feeding takes several hours of every day, but video recordings have shown that their perception of the time taken may be inaccurate.[7]

A team approach to the management of feeding problems in children with cerebral palsy

As a result of an increasing awareness of the prevalence and complexity of feeding problems in children with neurodevelopmental handicaps, a multidisciplinary team was established at Booth Hall Children's Hospital in 1989 to assess these problems (for a full description of this approach see Ref. 5).

Children are seen with their parents as day-cases in the assessment unit, with each child seen by all members of the team (Table 1).

The *speech therapist* first gathers information about the child's feeding and swallowing by taking a detailed feeding history and

Table 1. Team approach to swallowing disorders in children with neuro-developmental handicap

Core team:
- parents and carers
- speech therapist
- paediatric neurologist
- respiratory paediatrician
- paediatric gastroenterologist
- dietitian
- paediatric radiologist

examining oral structure and movement. She assesses current feeding skills by watching the parents feeding the child with their own utensils. Problems such as tongue thrust, oral hypersensitivity and the child's ability to cope with foods of different consistencies are identified at this stage.

The aims of the *paediatric neurologist's* assessment are to:

- identify specific symptoms such as dystonia and dyskinesia, which may contribute to the feeding difficulties;[5,8,21] and
- review the diagnosis and treatment of the underlying neurological disorder.

For example, extensor dystonia, which often passes unrecognised, can worsen feeding difficulties and cause stridor due to upper airway narrowing. It can be reduced by changing the child's sitting position during feeds.

The *respiratory paediatrician* assesses:

- whether the child has significant respiratory disease;
- the causes; and
- what treatment, if any, is needed.

A careful history is usually more rewarding than the examination, but a chest radiograph is performed to look for chronic inflammatory changes or persistent collapse of the lungs. It may be clear from the history that recurrent 'chest infections' are due to recurrent aspiration, and that it is not safe to persevere with oral feeding.

The *paediatric gastroenterologist* and the *dietitian* assess:

- the child's growth and nutritional status;
- the adequacy of the current diet; and
- whether there is any clinical evidence of GOR or oesophagitis.[23]

If severe GOR is suspected, or if insertion of a feeding gastrostomy is being planned, continuous 24-hour oesophageal pH monitoring will be arranged.

All children have a videofluoroscopic barium swallow performed by the *paediatric radiologist*. Although clinical assessment is vital, this is the only way to observe oropharyngeal function directly.[24-26] It enables oral control, bolus formation and propulsion, and the nature of the swallow reflex to be assessed.

Aspiration and, in those who aspirate, the presence and efficacy of a cough reflex can also be seen. The examination involves the parents and speech therapist who can describe the feeding difficulties and advise which foods should be tested. Swallowing is assessed with foods of different thicknesses and textures; liquids, rusks, yoghurt, cereals or chocolate buttons can all be opacified with barium.

Management

After the children have been seen by all the team, and the video-fluoroscopy recordings have been analysed, the neurologist and speech therapist explain the findings of the assessment to the parents and discuss what changes, if any, to feeding may be helpful (Tables 2 and 3). For some children, stabilising posture during feeds, with special adaptive seating or a soft cervical collar, or simple feeding equipment such as wide-bore straws may be recommended.

The speech therapist's assessment and the videofluoroscopy may suggest that avoidance of some textures and consistencies of food and an increase in the volume of others may facilitate swallowing and reduce the risk of aspiration.

The dietitian may suggest the introduction of nutritional supplements such as glucose polymers. A trial of thickening agents or prokinetic agents such as cisapride may be suggested if there is evidence of GOR, but medical treatment of this problem is often disappointing in children with cerebral palsy.[27]

If behavioural factors are thought to be contributing to the problems, a sensorimotor training programme can lead to improved tolerance and enthusiasm for eating in the child who has developed aversive reactions.

Table 2. Aims of feeding assessment in the handicapped child

Assess swallowing:
- history
- examination
- videofluoroscopy

Observe current feeding practice

Assess:
- nutritional status and growth
- respiratory problems
- underlying neurological problems

Table 3. Management of feeding disorders in cerebral palsy

Feeding:
- position (adaptive seating)
- equipment (wide-bore straws)
- texture/thickness of food
- supplements

Behaviour:
- jaw control
- sensorimotor training

Gastro-oesophageal reflux:
- thickeners
- cisapride

Enteral feeding:
- nasogastric feeds (short-term)
- gastrostomy ± fundoplication

Support and reassurance

Nasogastric feeding

Nasogastric feeding can be useful as a short-term measure to achieve adequate dietary intake, but repeated placement of the tube is distressing for the child and the appearance is often a cause of concern for the parents.

Gastrostomy feeding

Long-term gastrostomy feeding is now the established method of managing those children in whom oral feeding cannot achieve an adequate dietary intake, or where the risk of recurrent aspiration during feeding is unacceptably high, with little likelihood of improvement in the foreseeable future. It allows an adequate nutritional intake to be achieved and relieves carers and children of the burden of time-consuming and inefficient feeding. Many parents report a dramatic improvement in the quality of life of their child and the family after a gastrostomy feeding is started. Many children who require gastrostomy insertion also have severe GOR, so an antireflux procedure such as a Nissen or Boix-Ochoa fundoplication is performed in over half the children.[28]

Although gastrostomy feeding is a real advance for many children with severe cerebral palsy, it is not a risk-free panacea. Irrespective of which of the various techniques for gastrostomy insertion is used, there is a small but significant risk of morbidity—and indeed of mortality—associated with the procedure in this vulnerable group of patients. It is also important to recognise that, however difficult eating is in some of these children, the sensation of food can still be a source of pleasure that will be denied to them if they receive all their nutrition by a gastrostomy. This factor certainly influences some parents' decision about whether or not their child should have a gastrostomy inserted. A mixture of oral and gastrostomy feeding may be a reasonable compromise if there is not severe aspiration.

In some children, however, we are unable to suggest any improvements in the feeding practices that they have been using. We believe that reassuring the parents that what they are doing is safe and effective is often valuable for the family and other carers.

Conclusions

Feeding problems are common in children with cerebral palsy. They cause discomfort and distress to the children and their families, and result in inadequate nutrition, poor growth and recurrent respiratory illness.

Assessing feeding, nutrition and respiratory status is a time-consuming and complex process which is best carried out by a multidisciplinary team. Such an assessment can result in changes in feeding practices that significantly improve the quality of life of both child and carers. In the less severely affected child, simple measures such as better seating and equipment for feeding, or behavioural techniques to improve swallowing and reduce oral hypersensitivity, are often effective. In an increasing proportion of children with severe feeding difficulties, however, long-term gastrostomy feeding offers the best opportunity for achieving improved nutrition and growth, and for avoiding potentially life-threatening respiratory complications. Further research is needed to delineate precisely which children benefit most from such an approach, and to establish objectively the long-term benefits for children managed in this way.

The optimal method of assessing and managing these complex feeding difficulties remains unknown: different centres employ different approaches. It is beyond dispute, though, that each paediatric department caring for those with cerebral palsy should have an agreed policy for the investigation and management of this important, but often neglected, problem.

Acknowledgements

I am grateful for all that I have learnt from my fellow members of the Feeding and Swallowing Clinic at Booth Hall Children's Hospital, namely, Dr Michael Clarke, Ruth Miller, Alison Coates, Dr Adrian Thomas and Dr Rob Bisset.

References

1. Nolan C. *A damburst of dreams.* London: Weidenfeld and Nicolson, 1981: 9
2. Bax M. Eating is important. *Developmental Medicine and Child Neurology* 1989; **31**: 285–6
3. Jones PM. Feeding disorders in children with multiple handicaps. *Developmental Medicine and Child Neurology* 1989; **31**: 404–6
4. Reilly S, Skuse D. Characteristics and management of feeding problems of young children with cerebral palsy. *Developmental Medicine and Child Neurology* 1992; **34**: 379–88
5. Couriel JM, Bisset R, Miller R, Thomas A, Clarke M. Assessment of feeding problems in neurodevelopmental handicap: a team approach. *Archives of Disease in Childhood* 1993; **69**: 609–13
6. Stallings VA, Charney EB, Davies JC, Cronk CE. Nutrition-related growth failure of children with quadriplegic cerebral palsy. *Developmental Medicine and Child Neurology* 1993; **35**: 126–38
7. Reilly S, Skuse D, Poblete X. The prevalence of feeding problems in preschool children with cerebral palsy. *Developmental Medicine and Child Neurology* 1994; **36** (Suppl 70): 5–6
8. Logemann J. *Evaluation and treatment of swallowing disorders.* San Diego, CA: College-Hill Press, 1983
9. Dodds WD. The physiology of swallowing. *Dysphagia* 1989; **3**: 171–8
10. Kennedy JG, Kent RD. Physiological substrates of normal nutrition. *Dysphagia* 1988; **3**: 24–37
11. Editorial. Growth and nutrition in children with cerebral palsy. *Lancet* 1990; **i**: 1253–4
12. Stallings VA, Charney EB, Davies JC, Cronk CE. Nutritional status and growth of children with diplegic or hemiplegic cerebral palsy. *Developmental Medicine and Child Neurology* 1993; **35**: 997–1006
13. Spender QW, Charney EB, Stallings VA. Assessment of linear growth of children with cerebral palsy: use of alternative measures to height or length. *Developmental Medicine and Child Neurology* 1989; **31**: 206–14
14. Krick J, Murphy PE, Markham JFB, Shapiro BK. A proposed formula for calculating energy needs of children with cerebral palsy. *Developmental Medicine and Child Neurology* 1992; **34**: 481–7
15. Shapiro BK, Green P, Krick J, Allen D, Capute AJ. Growth of severely impaired children: neurological versus nutritional factors. *Developmental Medicine and Child Neurology* 1986; **28**: 729–33
16. Patrick J, Boland M, Stoski D, Murray GE. Rapid correction of wasting in children with cerebral palsy. *Developmental Medicine and Child Neurology* 1986; **28**: 734–9

17. Rempel GR, Colwell SO, Nelson RP. Growth in children with cerebral palsy fed via gastrostomy. *Pediatrics* 1988; **82**: 857–62
18. Logemann JA. Treatment for aspiration related to dysphagia: an overview. *Dysphagia* 1986; **1**: 34–8
19. Phelan PD, Landau LI, Olinsky A. Pulmonary complications of inhalation. *Respiratory illness in children.* Oxford: Blackwell, 1990: 234–49
20. Loughlin GM. Respiratory consequences of dysfunctional swallowing and aspiration. *Dysphagia* 1989; **3**: 126–30
21. Christensen JR. Developmental approach to pediatric neurogenic dysphagia. *Dysphagia* 1989; **3**: 131–4
22. Evans PM, Alberman E. Certified cause of death in children and young adults with cerebral palsy. *Archives of Disease in Childhood* 1991; **66**: 325–9
23. Booth IW. Silent gastro-oesophageal reflux: how much do we miss? *Archives of Disease in Childhood* 1992; **67**: 1325–7
24. Kramer SS. Radiologic examination of the swallowing impaired child. *Dysphagia* 1989; **3**: 117–25
25. Dodds WJ, Logemann JA, Stewart ET. Radiological assessment of abnormal oral and pharyngeal phases of swallowing. *American Journal of Radiology* 1990; **154**: 965–74
26. Dodds WJ, Stewart ET, Logemann JA. Physiology and radiology of the normal oral and pharyngeal phases of swallowing. *American Journal of Radiology* 1990; **154**: 953–63
27. Brueton MJ, Clarke GS, Sandhu B. Effect of cisapride on gastro-oesophageal reflux in children with and without neurological disorders. *Developmental Medicine and Child Neurology* 1990; **32**: 629–32
28. Spitz L, Roth K, Kiely EM, Brereton RJ, *et al.* Operation for gastro-oesophageal reflux associated with severe mental retardation. *Archives of Disease in Childhood* 1993; **68**: 347–51

14 Behavioural eating problems in young children

J E Douglas
*Consultant Clinical Psychologist, Department of Psychological
Medicine, Great Ormond Street Hospital for Children NHS Trust, London*

Feeding and eating problems in young children are common. One study has reported that over one-third of five year olds have mild to moderate eating or appetite problems.[1] Another study has shown that 16% of three year olds have a poor appetite and 12% are faddy.[2] In the paediatric population admitted to hospital with acute illness there have been estimates of between one and five per cent failing to thrive.[3]

Feeding difficulties in young children are major behavioural problems that can cause excessive and additional levels of stress in the families of children who have recovered from primary organic problems (eg following surgery for oesophageal atresia[4]) or with children who are still chronically ill (eg chronic renal failure,[5] oesophageal reflux[6]).

Data on the first 100 cases seen in our specialist behavioural feeding programme in an acute paediatric hospital (Great Ormond Street) are reported here; they have revealed a diversity in the range of problems treated, with referrals from eight hospital specialties including gastroenterology, surgery, ear, nose and throat, nephrology, cardiology, neurology, immunology and metabolic medicine. In this sample there were equal numbers of boys and girls, with a mean birth weight of 6.36 lb; 76% were full-term babies, with 7% born at less than 30 weeks gestation. Half the sample had received some special care after birth, 21% of them for more than four weeks.

Types of feeding problems

Different types of feeding difficulties can co-exist in the same child, providing a challenge to differentiate the problems. The emphasis in the literature on the dichotomy between organic and non-organic failure to thrive (FTT) has obscured the fact that many of these problems co-exist, and it is clinically far more relevant to try to identify the interrelationship between organic and psychosocial factors in the maintenance of the child's eating problem.[7] In one study of children hospitalised for FTT, 28% were diagnosed as organic, 46% non-organic and 26% of mixed aetiology.[8] This categorisation does not account for children who have a resolved organic condition which affected feeding experiences but who continue to have an eating problem.

FTT may or may not be associated with other types of feeding difficulties, so the emphasis on this diagnosis as the basis for treatment omits a large number of children with severe eating problems. In a sample of the first 100 cases seen in our unit, a primary problem could be classified in 85, but 15 children had several problems or a physical condition that had particular feeding issues. The 85 children with a primary problem could be subdivided into four groups (Table 1):

Eating inappropriate texture for age (n = 14)

Inappropriate textures of food for their age were being eaten by 44% of the sample. These children were either still on purée over the age of one year or had a mostly liquid diet, usually from a bottle, when they should have progressed to a full solid diet. All children in the programme were over one year old (mean age, 37 months) and were expected to be on a lumpy diet of soft and hard solids with finger foods. At referral, 42% were below the third centile for weight, but the remainder had their weight well maintained on the inappropriate textures. These children were not faddy—that is, they ate a full range of food types—but 71% were described by their parents as disinterested and frequently spitting out food (see Table 2).

Parents were concerned about the problem; they were faced with always liquidising their child's food or resorting to stage 1 baby foods, which made their child noticeably different from others of the same age and affected social functioning. In the children over the age of four years great concern was expressed about the school lunch difficulties.

Severe selective eating (n = 18)

Twenty-one per cent of the sample demonstrated severe selectivity or faddiness related to the range and types of food they were prepared to eat. Although most young children have food fads throughout their early years, the referred children were permanently highly selective. Some were eating only one type of food (eg chocolate biscuits) while others ate such a limited range of foods that they could never participate in normal family meals. Although 50% of the parents thought their child was underweight, none was

Table 1. Medical factors associated with eating problems in young children (n = 85)

Medical factor	Texture problem (%)	Faddy (%)	Failure to thrive (%)	Tube fed (%)
Have had operation	29	17	7	44*
ENT problems	43	22	14	26
GOR	29	6	21	56*
Allergies	21	33	14	31

* *p* = 0.05.
ENT = ear, nose and throat.
GOR = gastro-oesophageal reflux.

Table 2. Incidence of parent reported symptoms as a percentage of each type of feeding problem

Symptom	Texture problem (%) (n = 14)	Faddy (%) (n = 18)	Failure to thrive (%) (n = 14)	Tube fed (%) (n = 39)
Disinterest	71	61	86	62
Slow eater	50	39	64	33
Spits food	71	50	79	72
Poor weight gain	43	50	93*	59
Low quantity	100*	78	100*	90*
Faddy	0	94**	14	2
Gagging	57	56	36	49
Texture problem	100**	0	29	56**
Poor chewing	43	17	29	44
Involuntary vomiting	50*	11	14	36*

* *p* > 0.05.
** *p* = 0.000.

below the third percentile. These children were also unlikely to have a problem with the texture of the food (see Table 2).

The mean age of this group was significantly higher (52 months) than that of the children with other types of eating problems—which may have reflected the delay in parents being able to make this problem noticeable to their doctor. The mean age of onset (11 months) was also significantly later, reflecting the fact that the problems were related to behavioural conflicts with the parents rather than to aversive experiences for organic reasons (33% of these children had been subjected to force feeding). They were also less likely to have medical problems or a history of vomiting than children with other types of eating problems, although 33% had allergies and food sensitivities (see Table 1).

Failure to thrive (weight below the third percentile) (n = 14)

Thirty-six per cent of the sample were below the third percentile for weight, and 58% under the tenth. Interestingly, 58% of the sample had been poor feeders from birth, with 35% experiencing marked problems during this time, and 25% of these children were born at less than 30 weeks gestation.

The FTT children demonstrated chronic food refusal. Mothers described them as not caring about food, never asking for food, and never appearing to be hungry. They could miss meals with no noticeable signs. This problem started within the first three months of life in 77% of this group, and was therefore long-standing.

Parents had often been told to let their children starve in order to encourage them to eat. They may have tried this for one or two days but had then given in and provided milk or tempted the child with preferred foods. This technique had never worked in this sample of children. Nearly three-quarters of the FTT children had experienced tube feeding at some time in their lives in order to increase their weight, and 38% of the FTT children were still being tube fed when they started the programme. Over half the FTT children (56%) had experienced problems gaining weight even on tube feeds.

Tube feeding (n = 39)

Forty-two per cent of the total sample were being tube fed on referral, while 67% had been tube fed at some time in the past, 33% for longer than six months; 58% of those tube fed had shown good weight gain on tube feeds, but 42% had slow or inadequate weight gain. This group of children were varied on referral, with some accepting a low quantity of oral food or drink, and 36% totally refusing any oral feeding. The issue for all these children was to reduce their dependence on tube feeds by gradually increasing their oral intake and eventually to transfer them totally to oral feeding. Digestive, respiratory and cardiac complications appear to be the strongest predictors of a longer transition to oral feeding.[9] In this sample, 44% of the children had undergone operations—significantly more than in the other types of eating problems (see Table 1).

Over half (56%) the tube fed children had problems accepting normal textures for their age, but they were less likely to be faddy than the rest of the sample (Table 2), and 32% and 48% of them were below the third percentile for weight and height, respectively.

Difficult mealtime behaviour

Problems were experienced by 28% of the parents in getting their child to the table at mealtimes. This was because the child was either disinterested in food and did not want to eat or was worried and frightened by food and the prospect of eating. Some children were easily distracted, non-compliant and generally difficult to control, and their parents did not have the appropriate child management skills to persuade the child to sit quietly to eat. This problem did not exist on its own but was associated with other types of feeding difficulty.

Aetiology of feeding problems

In the last group of children a behavioural rather than an organic element was the primary consideration in the continuation of the feeding difficulty. This was not always the case, but children were accepted for treatment if it was thought that psychological intervention would ease the situation generally. A behavioural analysis of the feeding problem was therefore required rather than relying on an organic interpretation of the condition.

A learning theory approach was taken to attempt to understand the aetiology of the problems and provide some guidelines on the types of treatment approaches that would be most helpful. Two main themes in the children's history were relevant.

Early aversive experiences

Children who had early aversive experiences associated with feeding had developed phobic and avoidant reactions to food because of pain, nausea and distress experienced while feeding. (This has been called food aversion, and noted in other cases.[10,11]) Supporting this hypothesis have been the data collected on the frequency of choking, vomiting, gastro-oesophageal reflux (GOR) and force feeding experienced by the children.

At referral, 51% of the sample were choking or regurgitating, and 43% vomiting (72% had experienced significant vomiting), in 38% of them due to GOR. When past experiences of vomiting were examined, 47% had vomited four or more times daily, it had continued for six months or more in 42% of the sample (since the average age of these children was so young, this was a highly significant part of their total life experience in relation to eating), and 44% had received treatment for vomiting, either surgery or medication.

Some parents described always having a bowl under the high chair to catch the vomit at every mealtime; others reported excessive loads of washing and cleaning while their child vomited repeatedly each day. Some mothers were so conscientious that they tried to compensate for the lost food that had been vomited by feeding the child continuously throughout the day and were able to maintain a good weight gain despite excessive vomiting. This sometimes disguised the seriousness of the problem.

Children eating inappropriate textures or being tube fed were significantly more likely to have experienced vomiting that was frequent and medically treated than those with the other types of eating problems.

Other aversive experiences have been due to force feeding by parents, and 37% of the children had experienced minor force feeding. This included being fed against their will, shouted at and threatened, and being subjected to minor physical restraint. Another 14% had experienced major force feeding, in many instances continued for periods of several months, with their nose being held to make them swallow, their face slapped and their arms restricted in a towel or by the mother holding them in a tight grip while forcing the bottle into their mouth. Of the FTT children, 57% had experienced force feeding, 20% of them major force feeding.

Parents expressed great distress watching their child being force fed either by nursing staff or being made to do it themselves by health care professionals in the community.

Distortion of normal feeding experiences

Many of these children have experienced distortions of their normal developmental progression in feeding due to medical problems in the first year of life. Tube feeding for long periods in the first year of life and problems with weaning and introduction of lumpy solids have created stresses and distortions at significant developmental stages. Although tube feeding is used as a result of a feeding problem, it can at times compound or prolong the problem as the child or family may become dependent on the tube and be unable to transfer to oral feeding without considerable help and support.[10,12] The child may not have progressed through the normal eating stages and will therefore need to be weaned despite being much older. A child who has been unable to take any food orally for medical reasons will find the introduction of tastes and textures initially difficult and need a gentle and graded introduction to eating. Experiences of non-nutritive sucking and oral stimulation will often ease this transition.[13]

Another form of distorted experience is the prolongation of liquid or purée feeding beyond the end of the first year. There may be a critical time towards the end of the first year of life for the introduction of solids to an infant's diet.[14]

There were problems with weaning between three and six months in 66% of the sample, and in 37% the problems were marked; 53% of the children showed early refusal of spoon feeding, 36% of them marked refusal. The introduction of lumpy foods seemed to be a particularly difficult time, with parents commenting that their children weaned well on to purée but could not manage second-stage baby foods. Repeated attempts to get them to eat lumpy food failed. The child's resistance dominated the parents' behaviour to the extent that inappropriate textures were maintained for long periods of time.

Maintenance of childhood behavioural eating problems

Factors that maintain the child's eating problems may or may not be related to the aetiology of the problem. In some instances, the child's learnt experiences of aversion will maintain the problem. Thus, for example, GOR may have been successfully treated but the child still be afraid of food and eating. In other instances, the parents may need guidance, knowledge and structure about how best to feed their child orally. There may no longer be medical indications, but the child continues to lose weight whenever tube feeds are reduced because the parents have not learnt to provide high-calorie, low-quantity foods or have become dependent on the tube feeding to reduce their own level of anxiety about the child.

Parents' confidence in managing their child's behaviour can rapidly be undermined by acute or chronic ill health in their infant.

Overprotection, anxiety and depression are common features in parents who have experienced these traumas. This can further disrupt and undermine their management style.

Factors not associated with organic conditions can also occur and affect the child's eating pattern. Experiences of severe neglect or abuse may be revealed by significant FTT. Severe mental health problems in the parents may affect the development of an appropriate parent–child relationship which is responsive and reciprocal. Similarly, family or marital discord may adversely influence the child's or the parent's own emotional state (see Figure 1).

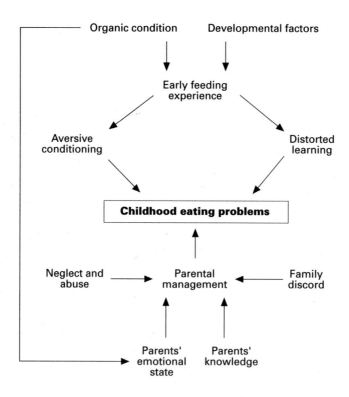

Fig. 1. *Factors that contribute to behavioural eating difficulties in young children*

Conclusion

Early childhood eating problems present a far more diverse pattern than has previously been reported. They cause considerable distress to parents and can take up a considerable amount of a paediatrician's time. In a proportion of children, several of these types of problems will co-exist, so their management and treatment can be complex and time-consuming. The paediatrician must therefore rely on a multidisciplinary team to manage these problems and assess the relative importance of behavioural and family issues in maintaining the problem. There are implications for the management of infants from the early months of life, throughout the course of a medical intervention or organic disorder and including the period when the child is considered medically recovered but still has an eating problem. The child has to learn how to eat, overcome fear and aversion, and the parents require support and direction how best to help their child have positive experiences with eating.

References

1. Butler NR, Golding J, eds. *From birth to five: a study of health and behaviour of Britain's five year olds.* London: Pergamon Press, 1986
2. Richman N, Stevenson J, Graham P. *Pre-school to school: a behavioural study.* London: Academic Press, 1982
3. Bithoney WG, Rathbun JM. Failure to thrive. In: Levine MD, Cary WB, Crocker AC, Gross RT, eds. *Developmental-behavioural paediatrics.* Philadelphia, PA: WB Saunders, 1983: 557–72
4. Puntis JWL, Ritson DG, Holden CE, Buick RG. Growth and feeding problems after repair of oesophageal atresia. *Archives of Disease in Childhood* 1990; **65**: 84–8
5. Ruley EJ, Bock GH, Kerzner B, Abbott AW, *et al.* Feeding disorders and gastro-oesophageal reflux in infants with chronic renal failure. *Pediatric Nephrology* 1989; **3**: 424–9
6. Harnsberger JK, Corey JJ, Johnson DG, Herbst JJ. Long term follow up of surgery for gastro-oesophageal reflux in infants and children. *Journal of Pediatrics* 1983; **102**: 505–8
7. Wittenberg JVP. Feeding disorder in infancy: classification and treatment considerations. *Canadian Journal of Psychiatry* 1990; **35**: 529–33
8. Homer C, Ludwig S. Categorisation of failure to thrive. *American Journal of Diseases of Children* 1981; **135**: 848–51
9. Bazyk S. Factors associated with the transition to oral feeding in infants fed by nasogastric tubes. *American Journal of Occupational Therapy* 1990; **44**: 1070–8
10. Handen BL, Mandell F, Russo DC. Feeding induction in children who refuse to eat. *American Journal of Diseases of Children* 1986; **140**: 52–4

11. Linscheid TR, Tarnowski KJ, Rasnake LK, Brams JS. Behavioral treatment of food refusal in a child with short gut syndrome. *Journal of Pediatric Psychology* 1987; **12**: 451–9

12. Geertsma MA, Hyams JS, Pelletier JM, Reiter S. Feeding resistance after parenteral hyperalimentation. *American Journal of Diseases of Children* 1985; **139**: 255–6

13. Field T, Ignatoff E, Stringer S, Brennan J, *et al.* Non-nutritive sucking during tube feedings: effects in pre-term neonates in an intensive care unit. *Pediatrics* 1982; **70**: 381–4

14. Illingworth RS, Lister J. The critical or sensitive period, with special reference to certain feeding problems in infants and children. *Journal of Pediatrics* 1964; **65**: 839–48

15 | Food intolerance

Timothy J David
Professor of Child Health, University of Manchester; Honorary
Consultant Paediatrician, University Department of Child Health, Booth Hall
Children's Hospital, Royal Manchester Children's Hospital and St Mary's
Hospital, Manchester

The subject of food intolerance is difficult and controversial. At one extreme are cases where multiple food intolerance has been inappropriately diagnosed, with resulting severe handicap.[1,2] At the other extreme are children with life-threatening and occasionally fatal reactions to foods.[3–6]

Definition of food intolerance

The first problem is to define the term 'food intolerance'. The best that can be done is to say that food intolerance is a 'reproducible adverse reaction to a specific food or food ingredient which is not psychologically based'. This definition is not without its difficulties, first because there is no definition of what constitutes an 'adverse reaction'. All eating can cause a reaction such as satiety, the urge to defecate, a feeling of warmth, or weight gain. Furthermore, families vary in their tolerance of events. For some, flatus is unacceptable and a problem, whereas for others it is the normal effect of eating baked beans. A second problem is that any food if taken in excess can cause adverse effects. For example, pears or honey are a rich source of fructose, which is relatively poorly absorbed compared with some other sugars. Excess fructose intake in small children can cause loose stools, particularly in certain predisposed individuals.[7,8] A third example is raised intracranial pressure as a result of vitamin A toxicity due to a high intake of chicken liver.[9] Finally, and perhaps the best known example, in susceptible subjects gout can result from an excessive intake of foods rich in purines.

The term 'intolerance' is preferred to 'allergy' when referring to adverse reactions to foods because it does not imply any particular mechanism. 'Food allergy' implies an immunological mechanism, which may be food-specific antibodies, immune complexes or cell-mediated reactions.

Prevalence of food intolerance

The most common foods leading to reports of intolerance in child-hood are cow's milk, eggs, nuts and fruit. However, the true preva-lence of food intolerance is unknown, and it has attracted little systematic study. It is said to be higher in infants than in adults, and it appears to be higher in atopic children than in non-atopic children. Food intolerance was reported in 19% of a sample of 866 children in Finland by the age of one year, 22% by two years, 27% by three years and 8% by six years.[10] In a prospective study of 480 children in the USA up to their third birthday, 16% were reported to have had reactions to fruit or fruit juice and 28% to other food.[11]

Natural history of food intolerance

Food intolerance is commonly reported in children, but studies show that it is usually of brief duration. For example, in the same US study,[11] although 28% of the 480 children had been reported to have food intolerance by the age of three years (80% of them by the age of 12 months), the offending food was back in the diet in half the children after only nine months and in virtually all (129 of 133) by the third birthday. Even severe reactions are not necessarily life-long, although the data here are rather limited. For example, Bock[12] reported nine children with very severe reactions to foods. Three were later able to tolerate normal amounts of the food, four to tolerate small amounts, and only two remained intolerant. The exception to this seems to be allergy to peanuts where the limited data available suggest that it is usually lifelong.[13]

Unreliability of parental reports

One practical difficulty is that the parents' reports are not always reliable. It is clear from studies in which parents' reports have been tested using double-blind challenges that parents' beliefs about food intolerance in their child are often wrong. In one study, parents' reports could be confirmed in only 37 (28%) of 133 children with reported food intolerance when the children were studied by double-blind food challenges;[11] in another study, only 27 (33%) of 81 reports of food intolerance in children could be confirmed by blind challenge.[14]

It becomes even more difficult to validate parents' reports of isolated reactions to food or food additives (reviewed in Ref. 5).

Lack of useful diagnostic or predictive tests

One practical difficulty in the management of suspected food intolerance in childhood is that simple and useful practical tests are not available. Skin prick and radio-allergosorbent tests (RAST), both of which look for specific IgE antibodies, and which give similar results, are unhelpful and not worth performing.[15] There are a large number both of false positive results (especially in children with atopic eczema) and of important false negative reactions. There are a number of reasons for the latter, but we (and others) have reported severe reactions to foods in the face of completely negative RAST tests.[4,16] Other difficulties with these tests are in the choice of extracts—the choice of a raw or cooked food is not straightforward—and that tests that look for IgE antibodies are not relevant to cases of non-IgE mediated reactions.

Double-blind placebo-controlled challenges

The best test to confirm or refute food intolerance is the double-blind placebo-controlled challenge, but at present this is mainly used as a research tool rather than a procedure for everyday clinical practice. Some of the best evaluated challenge materials have been freeze-dried foods in capsules,[17] but it is not practical to use these in small children who are unable to swallow capsules. This applies to most children with suspected food intolerance, given that most such cases are in children under the age of three years. Also, capsules are unacceptable to strictly observant orthodox Jewish patients because of the animal origin of gelatine. The alternative to capsules is either to disguise the test food in a carrier food, which is difficult and time-consuming even with a skilled dietitian, or to use a nasogastric tube, which is unpleasant and unpopular.

Another difficulty for double-blind challenges is when large or repeated doses of food are required, as in some cases of cow's milk protein intolerance, because reactions may occur only when larger quantities are taken. For example, Hill *et al* demonstrated that 8–10 g of cow's milk powder (corresponding to 60–70 ml of milk) was adequate to provoke an adverse reaction in some patients with cow's milk protein allergy, but others (with late-onset symptoms, particularly atopic eczema) required up to 10 times this volume of milk daily for more than two days before symptoms developed.[18] It is not easy to perform blind challenges with such large amounts of food. There can sometimes be problems with the route of administration. For example, adverse reactions to sulphites can be demonstrated only if they are given in solution; if given in capsule form, most subjects with sulphite intolerance do not react.

There are difficulties in the choice of food materials, in particular whether they should be raw or cooked. There is a preference for using raw foods, but this may increase the number of false positive results. For example, a number of children react to raw potato, but very few react to cooked potato. Conversely, a few individuals react only to a cooked food. As a generalisation, heating or cooking tends to reduce rather than increase the number of adverse reactions, with obvious implications for the effects of choosing a raw extract on the sensitivity and specificity of a challenge procedure.

An important confounding variable is the effect of disease activity. It is fairly well established in urticaria, and strongly suspected in atopic eczema, that certain subjects react to certain foods only when their disease is active, and can tolerate the food when it is inactive. It is commonly reported by parents of children with eczema that foods they cannot take at home in Britain without having quite marked adverse symptoms may be tolerated while on holiday in a sunny country. The reasons for improvement of atopic eczema while on holiday are not known.[19]

An additional major source of confusion is the possible additive effect of triggers. If this does occur (and it has never been proven for foods taken by mouth), there could be a situation in which, for example, a child would react adversely to bananas only if they were eaten at the same time as, say, apples and potatoes. If there is this additive effect, the accurate diagnosis of food intolerance is more complex. Clear evidence of such a phenomenon is demonstrated in patch testing in subjects with contact dermatitis,[20] and there is no doubt about an additive effect of non-food triggers. For example, there is a category of subjects who react adversely to food only on exercise—the so-called food-dependent exercise-induced anaphylaxis.[21] There are also certain subjects who react to foods only if they have recently taken aspirin.

Finally, there are statistical problems, which mean that a placebo-controlled challenge may have to be performed several times in an individual before being sure whether or not that subject is intolerant to a food.[5]

Food intolerance and atopic eczema

Despite the well recognised association between atopic eczema and food intolerance, there is a dearth of sound controlled trials to evaluate the benefit of dietary treatment. There are a number of possible approaches. One is to 'cut down' on one or two foods, but this type of tinkering is unhelpful, unlikely to succeed and, worst of all, at the end of such a trial the parents and physician are none the wiser whether or not food intolerance is relevant. A second option is to take a history and fully exclude foods for which there is a clear suggestion of intolerance. This approach is worth considering because there are children with a history of brisk reactions to certain foods (eg cow's milk protein) but where it is discovered that the parents are not in fact strictly avoiding this food; in this situation it may be worth finding out whether the child would benefit from complete exclusion of the food concerned. The next approach is a trial of milk and egg exclusion. There was some enthusiasm for this when it was first studied,[22] but subsequent work has not confirmed it as a useful approach.[23]

The lack of tests both to diagnose food intolerance and to predict which foods are or are not important means that any diet has to employ guesswork about likely trigger foods. A simple principle is that the more foods that are excluded the more likely there is to be benefit—if food intolerance is indeed important. As a result, in our unit a child whose eczema is severe enough to warrant an exclusion diet is started on a 'few-food' diet. This comprises lamb, potato, rice, a brassica (cabbage, cauliflower, brussels sprouts or broccoli), pear and tap-water. This is given for a six-week period, the rather long duration being for two reasons: first, the benefit of the diet may not be immediate; secondly, eczema is inherently a highly variable condition, and short periods of diets are likely to coincide with natural variation giving a misleading impression about whether or not the diet will be useful. It is important to use dietetic supervision for elimination diets to ensure complete avoidance of other foods, to make sure that the resulting diet is nutritionally adequate and also to give the parents practical help. At the end of the six-week period there is a decision-making assessment: if the diet is not markedly effective it can be abandoned, but if it is associated with notable improvement it can be continued, with the introduction, one by one, of all the foods that have been excluded, to enable identification of individual trigger foodstuffs.

Our initial impressions of this few-food diet were that it had an important place in the management of eczema. A study was then carried out in 63 children with severe atopic eczema, aged four months to 14.8 years, treated with a diet eliminating all but six foods for a six-week period.[24] Nine (14%) children abandoned the diet before the six weeks had elapsed, 21 (33%) completed the diet but did not benefit, and 33 (52%) obtained 20% or greater improvement in the disease severity score at six weeks—in these patients foods were reintroduced singly at weekly intervals. The outcome at

12 months was the same for the group who responded to the diet, the group who failed to respond, and the group who failed to comply, because of the tendency for eczema to improve markedly in all three groups.

Although dietary elimination of this type may be associated with immediate improvement, the long-term outcome therefore appears to be unaffected by dietary success or failure. The natural history of atopic eczema in childhood is of general improvement with age, and any short-term benefits of a diet have to be considered against a background of a lack both of data demonstrating long-term benefit from diets and of effect on the natural history of the condition. Further controlled studies are clearly needed, and are underway.

The ultimate diet—and also the ultimate test for food intolerance—is one in which the child takes no normal food or drink, not even tap-water, but consumes a so-called elemental diet. This is really a non-macromolecular diet, using amino acids and other ingredients which are unlikely to provoke an adverse reaction. We studied such a regimen in 37 children with severe atopic eczema, and showed that the use of an elemental diet, combined with being in hospital and stringent house-dust mite and pet avoidance measures, was associated with marked improvement in 27 (73%) of 37 subjects.[25] However, the study was uncontrolled, and it was impossible to tell how much the benefit was due to a placebo effect, how much to pet and house-dust mite avoidance and how much to food avoidance. A major practical problem is that in this and other studies the outcome of a diet could not be predicted on the basis either of the history or of investigations (eg RAST testing).

It has to be concluded that food is only one of many things that can trigger atopic eczema.[26] The history is not helpful in identifying which children will benefit from a diet, and unfortunately there is a lack of evidence that a diet affects the natural history of the condition. We still use few-food diets in children with atopic eczema, but now with rather less enthusiasm, confining this approach to the most severe cases, particularly those whose parents are keen to try a diet.

Placebo effects of diets

It is important to bear in mind that diets have a powerful placebo effect. This was well demonstrated, for example, in a study of dietary treatment of migraine. Salfield *et al* studied a diet which excluded vasoactive amines, and compared the results with a placebo high-fibre diet in 39 children with migraine.[27] The low amine diet was successful, reducing headaches from a mean of 13.8 over eight weeks to 7.5, and in 10 of the 19 children on this diet there was a 50% reduction in headaches. However, the control diet produced equally dramatic results: headaches fell from a mean of 13.3 to 6.9, and 11 of the 20 children on the placebo diet had a 50% reduction in headaches.

Elimination diet

Therapeutic principles of elimination diets

Given the lack of diagnostic tests, elimination diets in the context of food intolerance have to be considered as therapeutic trials. There are a number of basic principles. The first is to define the diet in terms of time, the duration required depending on the clinical problem. It is important to agree an end-point with the family, to re-assess the child at the end of the diet, and make sure that the diet is abandoned if it has not been helpful—otherwise, a child may remain indefinitely and needlessly on an elimination diet. If the diet is beneficial, it is important to employ planned reintroduction of foods singly, so that food triggers can be identified. This is often the most difficult aspect of the management, particularly in atopic eczema where there is considerable fluctuation in the severity of the disease from day to day and week to week. Flare-ups of the eczema may be due to natural variation in the condition, to an intercurrent infection, to teething or possibly to the food being tested. A food often has to be tried several times before it is possible to be sure whether or not it is a trigger. It must also be remembered that any improvement on a diet may simply be a coincidence or due to a placebo effect rather than to the avoidance of specific foods. It is helpful to use a dietitian in any elimination diet for the reasons given above.

Practical difficulties with elimination diets

There are a number of common practical difficulties with elimination diets in children. The major difficulty is that *unwrapped manufactured foods* are not labelled and therefore do not contain a list of ingredients. *Chocolate products* are a potential problem because they are covered by different food labelling regulations and are not required to list ingredients in the same way—though in practice they usually do. *Compound ingredients* are a practical difficulty. For example, it has to be declared on a tin of soup if it contains a sausage—but not what is in the sausage unless that sausage comprises more than a certain percentage of the total contents of the tin. *Flour* contains a number of permitted additives which do not have to be included on food labels, including soya protein which is present in almost all manufactured bread in the UK but is not usually declared as an ingredient on the food label. It is common to have reports of intolerance to *sesame seeds* when the problem is not the sesame seeds but the *egg glaze* used to hold the seeds in place on a bun. *Batter* should contain only flour and water but in practice sometimes contains cow's milk. With proper labelling, this should not be a problem.

Traces of protein in *oils* present a practical difficulty. A child who is allergic to *peanuts* should not receive peanut oil (also known as arachis oil or ground-nut oil, and unfortunately often described simply as 'vegetable oil'). Although the quantities of protein in the oil are low, they may be sufficient to cause problems in children who are very sensitive. So-called *vegetarian cheese* is another common problem. Parents of children with cow's milk protein intolerance often buy this, thinking that it is free from cow's milk protein, whereas the only difference between vegetarian and ordinary cheese is that the former is made with a non-animal source of rennet. Finally, *health food shops* are often a source of misinformation.[5,28]

Hazards of elimination diets

Elimination diets pose a number of potential hazards. The first is nutritional in that they may carry a risk of *calcium deficiency* in particular,[29,30] and there have been a number of reports of dietary deficiency as a result of elimination diets that were not properly supervised.[31–38] Diets may constitute a *handicap*; professionals may not realise what a burden it is to have a child who cannot eat a number of foods, particularly manufactured foods. There is evidence to show that elimination diets often pose a *financial burden*.[39] The *psychological effects* of diets have never been studied but it is unlikely that stopping small children from eating certain foods has no psychological sequelae. Finally, there is a real concern about the risk of *anaphylactic shock*, which is a problem for children with severe allergy to specific foods and is also a particular risk when treating children with stringent diets such as elimination diets.[4,16]

Food intolerance and asthma

Food is only one of many items which can provoke or worsen asthma, and it is an uncommon trigger of asthma in childhood.[40] In one careful study, food provoked asthma in only eight (6%) of 140 children with asthma.[41] It is uncommon for asthma to be the sole manifestation of food intolerance.[42] Food-provoked asthma is almost always accompanied by other symptoms (eg cutaneous or gastrointestinal). In one study, of eight children with food-provoked asthma, an offending food provoked other disorders in all of them (urticaria, 6; rhinitis, 2; eczema, 1).[41] In another study, the relevant food provoked other disorders in all 11 subjects (eczema, 8; urticaria, 7; vomiting, loose stools or abdominal pain, 4; rhinitis, 3).[43] Similarly, where other atopic disorders co-exist with asthma, the incidence of food intolerance is about four times higher than in children who have asthma alone.[41] A history that a food has already been observed to provoke asthma is almost always present in food-provoked asthma.[44] It is rare for it to escape the parents'attention, and in most cases they take steps to avoid the offending food without seeking medical advice.[45] As stated earlier, parents' histories of food intolerance in their children are often unreliable. In a study of children with asthma in whom the parents reported that one or more foods provoked asthmatic symptoms, double-blind challenges confirmed the parents' histories in only 11 (29%) of the 38 children and in only 14 (20%) of 70 challenges.[43]

The subject of food additives and asthma is reviewed in detail elsewhere.[5] Sulphite preservatives are fairly common potential triggers in children with asthma. The azo dyes tartrazine and ponceau, the non-azo dye eythrosine, the benzoate preservatives and monosodium glutamate are rare potential triggers. The suggestion that cola is a trigger is unproven and requires further investigation. Reactions to colouring agents or preservatives (other than sulphites) are an uncommon and overrated cause of clinically significant bronchoconstriction in children with asthma.

Behaviour problems and food intolerance

A childhood situation in which food or food additive intolerance is commonly suspected (but is usually not relevant) is when a child manifests behavioural problems. Management is complicated by the widespread belief amongst parents and some health professionals that food or food additives can have a major impact on children's behaviour. Repeated studies have failed to confirm this. For example, in one study 24 children (mean age 5.2 years) were studied with double-blind placebo-controlled challenges with tartrazine and benzoic acid (a preservative).[46] All the children gave a

history of immediate (within two hours) obvious adverse behavioural reaction to ingestion of tartrazine, and any lapse (ie any
ingestion of tartrazine) caused marked adverse behavioural symptoms. It was interesting to note that these children were on diets
excluding between two and 38 food items (mean, 23). Children who
currently had eczema or asthma as part of their reaction were
excluded from the study. Double-blind placebo-controlled challenges were performed in hospital using 50 mg and 250 mg
capsules, the contents of which were dissolved in pure orange juice.
The drink was given to the child by a nurse through an opaque
straw. Direct observations of the children showed that 18 of the 24
generally behaved normally whereas six had features of abnormal
behaviour. The result of this study was that there were no adverse
reactions either to placebo or to active substance; 22 children were
promptly returned to a normal diet without any problems, but the
parents of two children were unwilling to allow them to return to a
normal diet.

Conclusions

Some doctors hope that the current popular vogue for food intolerance, if ignored studiously enough, will go away. Others are inclined
to see reactions to food around every corner. But all doctors dealing
with children are confronted by parents who are concerned about
possible food or additive intolerance. Our understanding of why
some children are unable to tolerate certain foods, or of how they
often grow out of this intolerance, is poor. It is not known why
peanuts and fish are more capable of inducing violent reactions
than, say, lamb or potatoes. The molecular acrobatics that make one
antigen an allergen and another a non-allergen are not known.
Simplistic but unproven explanations abound.

This chapter has reviewed two extremes, atopic disease, where
food or food additive intolerance is sometimes important, and
behaviour problems, where food intolerance is widely overvalued.
Elimination diets should be seen as therapeutic trials, with clearly
defined end-points and dietetic supervision being important
ingredients.

References

1. David TJ. The overworked or fraudulent diagnosis of food allergy and
   food intolerance in children. *Journal of the Royal Society of Medicine* 1985;
   78 (Suppl 5): 21–31

2. Taylor DC. Outlandish factitious illness. In: David TJ, ed. *Recent advances in paediatrics*, vol. 10. London: Churchill Livingstone, 63–76
3. Patel L, Radivan FS, David TJ. Management of anaphylactic reactions to food. *Archives of Disease in Childhood* 1994; **71**: 370–5
4. David TJ. Anaphylactic shock during elimination diets for severe atopic eczema. *Archives of Disease in Childhood* 1984; **59**: 983–6
5. David TJ. *Food and food additive intolerance in childhood.* Oxford: Blackwell, 1993
6. Sampson HA, Mendelson L, Rosen JP. Fatal and near-fatal anaphylactic reactions to food in children and adolescents. *New England Journal of Medicine* 1992; **327**: 380–4
7. Kneepkens CMF, Jakobs C, Douwes AC. Apple juice, fructose, and chronic nonspecific diarrhoea. *European Journal of Pediatrics* 1989; **148**: 571–3
8. Wales JKH, Primhak RA, Rattenbury J, Taylor CJ. Isolated fructose malabsorption. *Archives of Disease in Childhood* 1989; **65**: 227–9
9. Mahoney CP, Margolis MT, Knauss TA, Labbe RF. Chronic vitamin A intoxication in infants fed chicken liver. *Pediatrics* 1980; **65**: 893–6
10. Kajosaari M. Food allergy in Finnish children aged 1 to 6 years. *Acta Paediatrica Scandinavica* 1982; **71**: 815–9
11. Bock SA. Prospective appraisal of complaints of adverse reactions to foods in children during the first 3 years of life. *Pediatrics* 1987; **79**: 683–8
12. Bock SA. Natural history of severe reactions to foods in young children. *Journal of Pediatrics* 1985; **107**: 676–80
13. Bock SA, Atkins FM. The natural history of peanut allergy. *Journal of Allergy and Clinical Immunology* 1989; **83**: 900–4
14. May CD, Bock SA. A modern clinical approach to food hypersensitivity. *Allergy* 1978; **33**: 166–88
15. David TJ. Conventional allergy tests. *Archives of Disease in Childhood* 1991; **66**: 281–2
16. David TJ. Hazards of challenge tests in atopic dermatitis. *Allergy* 1989; **44** (Suppl 9): 101–7
17. Bock SA, Sampson HA, Atkins FM, Zeiger RS, *et al.* Double-blind, placebo-controlled food challenge (DBPCFC) as an office procedure: a manual. *Journal of Allergy and Clinical Immunology* 1988; **82**: 986–97
18. Hill DJ, Ball G, Hosking CS. Clinical manifestations of cow's milk allergy in childhood. I. Associations with *in vitro* cellular immune responses. *Clinical Allergy* 1988; **18**: 469–79
19. Turner MA, Devlin J, David TJ. Holidays and atopic eczema. *Archives of Disease in Childhood* 1991; **66**: 212–5
20. McLelland J, Shuster S. Contact dermatitis with negative patch tests: the additive effect of allergens in combination. *British Journal of Dermatology* 1990; **122**: 623–30
21. Kidd JM, Cohen SH, Sosman AJ, Fink JN. Food-dependent exercise-induced anaphylaxis. *Journal of Allergy and Clinical Immunology* 1983; **71**: 407–11
22. Atherton DJ, Sewell M, Soothill JF, Wells RS, Chilvers CED. A double-blind controlled crossover trial of an antigen-avoidance diet in atopic eczema. *Lancet* 1978; **i**: 401–3

23. Neild VS, Marsden RA, Bailes JA, Bland JM. Egg and milk exclusion diets in atopic eczema. *British Journal of Dermatology* 1986; **114**: 117–23

24. Devlin J, David TJ, Stanton RHJ. Six food diet for childhood atopic dermatitis. *Acta Dermato-Venereologica* 1991; **71**: 20–4

25. Devlin J, David TJ, Stanton RHJ. Elemental diet for refractory atopic eczema. *Archives of Disease in Childhood* 1991; **66**: 93–9

26. David TJ, Devlin J, Ewing CI. Atopic and seborrheic dermatitis: practical management. *Pediatrician* 1991; **18**: 211–7

27. Salfield SAW, Wardley BL, Houlsby WT, Turner SL, *et al.* Controlled study of exclusion of dietary vasoactive amines in migraine. *Archives of Disease in Childhood* 1987; **62**: 458–60

28. David TJ. The unhealthy nature of health foods. *Maternal and Child Health* 1990; **15**: 228–30

29. David TJ, Waddington E, Stanton RHJ. Nutritional hazards of elimination diets in children with atopic eczema. *Archives of Disease in Childhood* 1984; **59**: 323–5

30. Devlin J, Stanton RHJ, David TJ. Calcium intake and cow's milk free diets. *Archives of Disease in Childhood* 1989; **64**: 1183–4

31. Editorial. Exotic diets and the infant. *British Medical Journal* 1978; **i**: 804–5

32. Lloyd-Still JD. Chronic diarrhea of childhood and the misuse of elimination diets. *Journal of Pediatrics* 1979; **95**: 10–3

33. Roberts IF, West RJ, Ogilvie D, Dillon MJ. Malnutrition in infants receiving cult diets: a form of child abuse. *British Medical Journal* 1979; **i**: 296–8

34. Tripp JH, Francis DEM, Knight JA, Harries JT. Infant feeding practices: a cause for concern. *British Medical Journal* 1979; **ii**: 707–9

35. Tarnow-Mordi WO, Moss C, Ross K. Failure to thrive owing to inappropriate diet free of gluten and cow's milk. *British Medical Journal* 1984; **289**: 1113–4

36. Hughes M, Clark N, Forbes L, Colin-Jones DG. A case of scurvy. *British Medical Journal* 1986; **293**: 366–7

37. Labib M, Gama R, Wright J, Marks V, Robins D. Dietary maladvice as a cause of hypothyroidism and short stature. *British Medical Journal* 1989; **298**: 232–3

38. Dagnelie PC, van Staveren WA, Hautvast JG. Stunting and nutrient deficiencies in children on alternative diets. *Acta Paediatrica Scandinavica* 1991; **374** (Suppl): 111–8

39. Macdonald A, Forsythe WI. The cost of nutrition and diet therapy for low-income families. *Human Nutrition Applied Nutrition* 1986; **A40**: 87–96

40. Bock SA. Food-related asthma and basic nutrition. *Journal of Asthma* 1983; **20**: 377–81

41. Novembre E, Martino M, Vierucci A. Foods and respiratory allergy. *Journal of Allergy and Clinical Immunology* 1988; **81**: 1059–65

42. Novembre E, Veneruso G, Sabatini C, Bonazza P, *et al.* Incidenza dell'asma da allergia alimentare in eta pediatrica. *Pediatria Medica e Chirurgica* 1987; **9**: 399–404

43. May CD. Objective clinical and laboratory studies of immediate hypersensitivity reactions to foods in asthmatic children. *Journal of Allergy and Clinical Immunology* 1976; **58**: 500–15

44. Onorato J, Merland N, Terral C, Michel FB, Bousquet J. Placebo-controlled double-blind food challenge in asthma. *Journal of Allergy and Clinical Immunology* 1986; **78**: 1139–46

45. Hill LW. Food sensitivity in 100 asthmatic children. *New England Journal of Medicine* 1948; **238**: 657–9

46. David TJ. Reactions to dietary tartrazine. *Archives of Disease in Childhood* 1987; **62**: 119–22

16 | Home parenteral nutrition

W Michael Bisset
*Senior Lecturer in Child Health, Department of Child Health,
University of Aberdeen*

A steady intake of food and absorption of nutrients is required for growth and development to proceed normally in every child. If gastrointestinal function is severely compromised by disease, the supply of nutrients is reduced and intravenous nutrition may be the only means by which the normal health of the child can be maintained. When intravenous nutrition was first introduced into paediatrics there was a high rate both of septic and of metabolic complications and, as a consequence, patients requiring long-term therapy often died. Over the last 20 years, with improvements in the design of parenteral feeding regimes and in the care and insertion techniques of central venous catheters, it is now possible to maintain children on intravenous nutrition for many years; this has resulted in many children spending prolonged periods in hospital receiving this treatment.[1-4]

Programmes for discharge from hospital and treatment at home of children requiring parenteral nutrition first appeared from the USA and France in the early 1980s.[5,6] In many ways, Britain has been slow to develop this therapy. This chapter describes the experience of one centre, the Hospital for Sick Children, Great Ormond Street, London, in the selection, training, discharge and follow-up of 20 children who required parenteral nutrition.

Indications for home parenteral nutrition

Any child who is dependent on parenteral nutrition and who does not require complex nursing support should be considered for this treatment. To many, prolonged intravenous therapy at home seems an unreasonable burden to place on any parent, but it has been shown that most parents are able to care competently for their child and that any burden placed upon them is likely to be less than if their child were still in hospital.

The majority of children discharged home on parenteral nutrition have suffered severe gastrointestinal disease (Table 1), although more recently this treatment has been used for children with both malignant disease and AIDS.

Children with gastrointestinal disease may be divided into three main groups:

- short gut syndrome;
- neuropathic or myopathic disease of the gut leading to the development of intestinal pseudo-obstruction; and
- intractable diarrhoea of infancy.

While it may be technically possible to support any child, irrespective of the underlying disease, this may not always be desirable. The success of the treatment in a well organised centre is related, first, to the ability of the parents to cope with the management of their child and, second, to the severity of the gastrointestinal disease. In many children, particularly those with short gut syndrome,

Table 1. Common indications for home parenteral nutrition

Gastrointestinal disease

- Reduced length of gut

    Intestinal resection
        Necrotising enterocolitis
        Volvulus
        Multiple intestinal atresia
        Crohn's disease
    Congenital short intestine

- Motility disturbance

    Myopathic pseudo-obstruction
    Neuropathic pseudo-obstruction
    Hirschprung's disease involving small intestine

- Intractable diarrhoea of infancy

    Congenital enteropathy
    Auto-immune enteropathy
    Congenital secretory diarrhoea

Systemic disease

- Malignant disease
- Acquired immune deficiency syndrome

the adaptive response of the residual gut may take over a year; if the child can be supported through this period, the outcome is likely to be good. In contrast, where there is evidence of progressive disease or a failure of adaptation, such as might occur with AIDS, the outcome is likely to be poor.

Administration of home parenteral nutrition

It is essential that a reliable means of venous access be secured. Traditionally, a surgically inserted Hickman-Broviac type of catheter has been used for prolonged parenteral nutrition.[7] If the line is inserted with full aseptic precautions with the tip placed in the right atrium, the risk of complications from both sepsis and venous thrombosis is reduced. More recently, infusion ports such as the Port-a-cath have been used for parenteral nutrition. These have the advantage that the device is hidden under the skin, but the disadvantage that a needle stick is required prior to each use. Irrespective of which type of catheter is used, prolonged use can be expected where the standard of care is high.

It is usual for home parenteral nutrition to be administered for 12 hours overnight using an accurately calibrated and alarmed volumetric infusion pump. This allows the child to be free from the infusion to attend school and otherwise live a normal life. If the child has residual intestinal function that allows a significant oral intake, it may be possible to give the parenteral nutrition on only five or six nights per week. This allows the child and the parents greater freedom of movement.

Where possible, attempts are made to formulate the home parenteral nutrition solution as an 'all in one bag', which simplifies the regime by requiring only one infusion pump. It is important always to maintain as much enteral nutrition in the child as possible, as this may not only be helpful in preventing vitamin and trace metal deficiencies but also speed up the rate at which the gut adapts and reduce the risk of liver disease developing. For some children in whom all the nutrients have to be given intravenously, it is likely that the parents may have to make additions to this solution (ie intravenous vitamins). This will not only increase the workload for the parents but also increase the risk of introducing infection.

Organisation

It is a major undertaking to send a child home on parenteral nutrition, not only for the child's family but also for the medical and nursing staff who will support the child.[8,9] Guidelines drawn up in a report published by the King's Fund[10] suggest that patients should be sent home on parenteral nutrition only when the hospital has a well organised nutrition team, extensive experience in parenteral nutrition and the facilities to train the patients and their parents. In addition, the hospital should be able to support the treatment of the patient at home through liaison with the child's general prac- titioner (GP) and the community team, and be in a position to provide a 24-hour advisory service. The report also considers it important that financial arrangements should not hinder the prompt discharge of a patient who could receive parenteral nutri- tion at home.

There are several major obstacles that prevent the discharge of children home on parenteral nutrition. First, there is a reluctance by caring professionals to recognise that the parents might be capa- ble of carrying out complicated medical treatment at home. Results from follow-up studies both in the UK and abroad have, however, clearly shown that most parents are capable of carrying out this treatment—indeed, morbidity and mortality are reduced on discharge home. Second, the present funding structure within the National Health Service (NHS) makes it difficult to organise expen- sive medical care in the community. It has been estimated that it costs about £30,000 per year to maintain a child at home on par- enteral nutrition, while the same child in hospital may cost up to £100,000 per year, but, as treatment at home is likely to be funded from a different source, this is often seen as a *new* burden rather than as an overall financial saving to the country. Most children on home parenteral nutrition (of whom there are probably about 50 in the UK at present) have their therapy arranged in an *ad hoc* manner. Where possible, the parenteral nutrition solutions are prescribed by the GP on an FP10 form, and funding is sought from the local com- munity paediatric budget (if it exists) to provide the infusion pump and consumables. This system is cumbersome and it would be preferable if central funding were available for the provision of expensive therapies in the community. Such funding exists in France; in the USA, where the majority of treatment is funded by medical insurance, the financial saving of home treatment is well recognised and financial obstacles to the provision of home par- enteral nutrition are fewer.

The majority of children on home parenteral nutrition in the UK are supplied by commercial home care companies who are able to arrange for the formulation and delivery of the parenteral nutrition solutions and the supply of all consumable items that may be required. In addition, these companies are able to provide round the clock servicing of infusion pumps and generally provide a standard of service that many NHS hospitals or trusts would find difficult to match.

Close liaison is required between the hospital, the child's GP and community nurses. The social services and education departments and other relevant organisations should be aware of the child's problems and be in a position to offer support. In addition, support groups for parents looking after children on home parenteral nutrition exist and are of great benefit to the parents.

Outcome of treatment

In a recent study from the Hospital for Sick Children, Great Ormond Street, 20 children on home parenteral nutrition were followed for a total of 48 patient-years (the patient details are shown in Table 2). One patient died during the initial follow-up period following the attempted vascular reconstruction of her gut. Subsequently, over the last 18 months, three more of these children have died, two from sepsis and one from pulmonary embolus. Of the remaining 16, one has had a successful gut transplantation and four have now been able to discontinue their total parenteral nutrition. Five of the 11 still on parenteral nutrition are showing increasing enteral food tolerance with time. As with other studies, it was found that the children grew and developed normally.[11]

Complications of treatment

The main complications of treatment relate to the central line.[12,13] The results in the 20 children were compared during their time in hospital and the subsequent period at home (Table 3). The startling and unexpected findings were that the average life of a central

Table 2. Details of children discharged from hospital on home parenteral nutrition.[1,4]

20 children	16 UK
	4 overseas
Age of discharge	4 months to 15 years
Follow-up	9 months to $6\frac{1}{2}$ years
Total follow-up	48 patient-years at home
	28 patient-years in hospital

Table 3. Central line survival and infection at home and in hospital in a consecutive series of 20 children from the Hospital for Sick Children, London (total follow-up, 48 patient-years)

	Hospital	Home
Infection rate	1 in 142 days	1 in 567 days
Average line life	175 days	567 days

venous catheter at home was three times longer than in hospital and that central line infections were four times more likely in hospital. These figures have been mirrored in almost every other published study of home parenteral nutrition, and clearly show that the risk of line-related complications is greatly reduced by discharging the children home to their parents, where the standard of care is likely to be better than in most hospitals. It was also interesting to note that there was no difference in the type of bacterial infection between the home and hospital group and that loss of the ileocaecal valve did not predispose patients to higher sepsis rates. Central venous thrombosis, another complication which can develop during prolonged parenteral nutrition,[14] may be more common in those patients who have more frequent episodes of sepsis.

The other main group of complications relate to nutritional deficiencies. In three of the 20 children in the study neurological symptoms developed as a consequence of problems of compliance with the administration of water-soluble vitamins, and one child became hypothyroid from iodine deficiency. All deficiencies were corrected without serious ill effect. Cholestasis and cholethiasis are well recognised complications of prolonged parenteral nutrition,[15] but by ensuring that all patients maintained some enteral intake and by keeping sepsis levels as low as possible, these complications were uncommon. In three patients discharged home with cholestatic jaundice the improved care provided by their parents led to increased enteral intake and reduced sepsis, with resulting resolution of their icterus.[16]

Conclusion

Home parenteral nutrition has been successfully developed in a number of centres in the UK over the last ten years. It has consistently been shown that children grow and develop normally on this treatment, and that it can be provided at reduced cost and increased safety in the comfort of the patient's own home. The quality of life of both the child and the family is, as a consequence, improved. For the child unfortunate enough to suffer from severe intestinal failure, home parenteral nutrition at present offers the best prospects for survival—which it is likely to continue until the outcome of gut transplantation significantly improves.

Despite the apparent success of this form of treatment, the funding and prompt provision of therapy remain a financial and administrative minefield and must surely be depriving some children of the chance of a more normal life at home.

References

1. Bisset WM, Stapleford P, Long S, Chamberlain A, *et al.* Home parenteral nutrition in chronic intestinal failure. *Archives of Disease in Childhood* 1992; **67**: 109–14

2. Amarnath RP, Fleming CR, Perrault J. Home parenteral nutrition in chronic intestinal diseases: its effect on growth and development. *Journal of Pediatric Gastroenterology and Nutrition* 1987; **6**: 89–95

3. Dahlstrom KA, Strandvik B, Kopple J, Ament ME. Nutritional status in children receiving home parenteral nutrition. *Journal of Pediatrics* 1985; **107**: 219–24

4. Bisset WM, Meadows NJ. Home parenteral nutrition in children. In: Kirschner B, Walker-Smith JA, eds. *Paediatric gastroenterology: clinical paediatrics.* London: Baillière Tindall, 1994; **2**: 705–22

5. Cannon RA, Byrne MJ, Ament ME, Gates B. Home parenteral nutrition in infants. *Journal of Pediatrics* 1980; **96**: 1098–104

6. Gorski AM, Goulet O, Lamor M, Postaire M, *et al.* Nutrition parentérale à domicile chez l'enfant. Bilan de 8 ans d'activité chez 88 malades. *Archives Françaises de Pédiatrie* 1989; **46**: 323–9

7. Pokorny WJ, Black CT, McGill CW, Splaingard ML, *et al.* Central venous catheters in older children. *American Surgeon* 1987; **53**: 524–7

8. Berry RK, Jorgensen S. Growing with home parenteral nutrition: adjusting to family life and child development. *Pediatric Nursing* 1988; **14**: 43–5

9. Berry RK, Jorgensen S. Growing with home parenteral nutrition: maintaining a safe environment. *Pediatric Nursing* 1988; **14**: 155–7

10. Lennard-Jones JE, ed. *A positive approach to nutrition as treatment.* London: King's Fund Centre, 1992

11. Ralston CW, O'Connor MJ, Ameny M, Berquist W, Parmalee AH. Somatic growth and developmental functioning in children receiving prolonged home total parenteral nutrition. *Journal of Pediatrics* 1984; **105**: 842–6

12. Ladefoged K, Efsen F, Christoffersen JK, Jarnum S. Longterm parenteral nutrition. II. Catheter-related complications. *Scandinavian Journal of Gastroenterology* 1981; **16**: 913–9

13. Rannem T, Ladefoged K, Tvede M, Lorentzen JE, Jarnum S. Catheter-related septicaemia in patients receiving home parenteral nutrition. *Scandinavian Journal of Gastroenterology* 1986; **21**: 455–60

14. Graham L, Gumbiner CH. Right atrial thrombosis and superior vena cava syndrome in a child. *Pediatrics* 1984; **73**: 225–9

15. Roslyn JL, Berquist WE, Pitt HA, Mann LL, *et al.* Increased risk of gallstones in children receiving total parenteral nutrition. *Pediatrics* 1983; **71**: 784–9

16. Cohen C, Olsen MM. Pediatric total parenteral nutrition: liver histopathology. *Archives of Pathology and Laboratory Medicine* 1981; **105**: 152–6

PART FOUR

National and international issues of nutrition

17 | Educational challenges

Anthony F Williams
Senior Lecturer and Consultant in Neonatal Paediatrics, St George's Hospital Medical School, London

Nutritional state during growth and development has far-reaching health consequences which extend into adult life, so the science of nutrition has greater relevance to paediatrics and its subspecialties than to most other areas of medicine. From a preventive standpoint, childhood diseases of primarily nutritional aetiology are still common (eg iron deficiency) and the prevalence of some is increasing (eg obesity). From a therapeutic standpoint, the importance of diet in clinical management is increasingly recognised. Despite considerable advances in genetics and tissue transplantation, diet remains the mainstay of treatment for the commoner inborn errors of metabolism. Moreover, it is becoming clear that nutritional assessment and provision of appropriate dietetic support influence outcome in both acute and chronic childhood disorders.

Despite its importance, nutrition has been a neglected aspect of medical education. The King's Fund Centre report, *A positive approach to nutrition as treatment*,[1] published in 1992, stated:

> Clinical nutrition was not taught to the present generation of doctors and it is still a Cinderella subject in undergraduate medical schools. Teaching has lagged behind nutritional research which has forged ahead, so increasing the gap between knowledge and practice.

Research continues to expand the already large body of knowledge related to paediatric nutrition. Indeed, nutrition constituted the primary topic of 12% of peer reviewed papers published in three major European paediatric journals in 1991–92.[2] The White Paper, *The health of the nation*,[3] has emphasised further the potential contribution of optimal nutrition to disease prevention both in childhood and in adult life. The Nutrition Task Force, established by the Department of Health (DoH) to advise ministers on action required to meet dietary and nutritional targets set out in *The health of the nation*, highlighted a need to improve nutrition education among health professionals. It has published a *Core curriculum for nutrition in the education of health professionals*,[4] which calls for the integration of nutrition education into the overall training of *all* health professionals.

Meeting the challenge to integrate nutrition education into paediatric training demands the identification of current obstacles, the clarification of learning objectives, and implementation.

Obstacles to nutrition education

What is nutrition?

Nutrition can be hard to define as an academic discipline; it cuts across the conventional subject areas of the preclinical and clinical curricula. It can neither be characterised by a specific methodology (cf molecular biology) nor be easily integrated into medical specialties conventionally based (for historical reasons) around anatomical systems rather than physiological functions.

The late Egon Kodicek remarked that nutrition is distinguished by the question being posed rather than by the methodology employed;[5] finding the answer involves a host of 'conventional' preclinical and clinical disciplines from molecular biology to epidemiology, and from respiratory physiology to sociology.

Another definition of the science of nutrition is:

> . . . the sum of the processes concerned with the growth, maintenance and repair of the living body as a whole, or its constituent parts.[6]

Such an ambitious definition, however, comprising almost the whole of human biology, perhaps obscures rather than clarifies the application of nutrition to clinical paediatrics. The term 'nutrition' may possibly be best defined as the study of the effects of diet and dietary constituents on the development, structure and function of the organism.

Where does nutrition fit into a medical career?

Doctors embarking on a career in paediatrics tend to orientate towards subspecialty career goals. For example, they recognise the position of paediatric cardiologist or paediatric neurologist, and can follow clearly defined pathways of training leading to eventual consultant appointment. Failure to recognise clinical nutrition as a paediatric subspecialty in the UK both damages motivation to learn and militates against provision of organised training.

Nutrition as a branch of therapeutics?

It has been argued that nutrition is a pure academic discipline and that the application of nutritional science is more appropriately termed 'dietetics'. Parallels can then be drawn between pharmacology/clinical pharmacology and nutrition/dietetics. Since clinical pharmacology and dietetics are effectively branches of therapeutics, McLaren has argued for the appointment of 'dietetic physicians' as the counterparts of clinical pharmacologists.[7]

Nevertheless, an important difference exists between nutrition and pharmacology as they are applied to medicine. Nutrition extends beyond the boundaries of therapy to disease prevention and health promotion. In this context, promoting a healthy diet involves changing the behaviour of children and their families; this requires a different approach to the usual medical diagnosis/treatment prescription model. If knowledge is to be put into practice, training in nutrition clearly needs to be accompanied by tuition in effective methods of health promotion and behavioural modification.

Time for teaching nutrition

The explosion of scientific knowledge in all areas of medicine puts pressure on the availability of time to teach nutrition. This is compounded by a philosophical shift away from core teaching to self-selected modules at undergraduate level and an anticipated reduction in the period of specialist postgraduate training leading to consultant appointment. Lack of time must not be viewed as an excuse for neglecting nutrition but as a strong stimulus to define learning objectives and curricula appropriate to each level of training. This will permit integration of nutrition into the curriculum.

Wider application of nutritional science in paediatrics is crucial to both the prevention and treatment of childhood disease. It seems paradoxical that a discipline with such major implications has not hitherto been granted the status of a curriculum or recognition as a paediatric subspecialty in its own right.

Learning objectives

General objectives

The objectives of nutrition education in the education of health professionals have been set out by the Nutrition Task Force:[4]

1. To appreciate the importance and relevance of nutrition to health promotion and the prevention of disease.
2. To understand the basic scientific principles of human nutrition.
3. To recognise nutrition-related problems in individuals and in the community.

4. To give consistent and sound dietary advice and make appropriate referral to a state registered dietitian.

5. To know and be able to promote and explain current dietary recommendations including the advantages of breast feeding.

6. To provide appropriate and safe clinical nutritional support and to know when and how to refer to a state registered dietitian.

7. To understand the relative costs and benefits of nutritional measures compared with other approaches to preventive and therapeutic care.

8. To assess the validity of nutritional scientific literature and media reports.

Objectives specific to paediatrics

Paediatricians in training should be able to see how these general objectives can be applied to clinical cases. An example is to consider what could be learnt from treating a child with iron deficiency (the numbers refer to the general objectives listed above):

1. epidemiology of iron deficiency (prevalence and risk factors); cultural and socio-economic influences on diet.

2. defining dietary iron requirements (interpreting the lower reference and reference nutrient intakes for iron[8]);
physiological functions of iron;
factors determining iron stores and iron distribution;
factors affecting bioavailability of dietary iron;
factors increasing iron loss (bleeding, gastrointestinal infection).

3. definition of iron deficiency (diagnostic criteria);
methods of dietary assessment;
clinical effects of iron deficiency;
recognition of diet-related problems associated with iron deficiency;
consideration of screening for iron deficiency.

4. advice about appropriate dietary change in iron deficiency;
problems associated with changing diet and methods of overcoming these.

5. philosophy underlying current infant feeding advice directed at prevention of iron deficiency (prolonging breast feeding, avoidance of cow's milk, vitamin C, etc);
reasons for failure to follow advice;
strategies for changing behaviour.

7. relative benefits of pharmacological approach (iron supplements) or dietary approach (changing eating behaviour) to treatment.

8. using knowledge accrued, be able to interpret research literature and suggest future research directions;
   interpret critically the nutritional claims made for infant formula and other dietetic products in improving iron status.

Learning objectives and career stage

Nutrition education also needs to be integrated into the curriculum vertically. The major vertical divisions in paediatric training are shown in Table 1. The curriculum at each level will vary both in scope and in depth of knowledge. Education in paediatric nutrition at undergraduate level needs to build on the basic scientific principles of human nutrition taught in most medical schools as part of the biochemistry and physiology curricula.

The main aims of teaching during the undergraduate paediatric course should be to:

- show how nutritional requirements and patterns of eating change during development;

- indicate the importance of nutrition in the prevention of disease; and

- highlight the social and cultural importance of dietetics as an aspect of paediatric medical therapy.

The Standing Committee on Nutrition (SCN) of the British Paediatric Association (BPA) has produced a core curriculum for training medical undergraduates in paediatric nutrition (available as a BPA pamphlet[9]). More recently, the SCN has considered the post-basic nutrition training of doctors specialising in paediatrics. A curriculum (see Appendix) has been produced which will be incorporated into curricula for general professional training in paediatrics and child health and, where indicated, into higher specialist training programmes. It reveals the scope of nutrition in paediatrics,

Table 1. Levels of training at which nutrition education needs to be integrated

Paediatric training	Professional level
Basic education	Undergraduate
General professional training	Senior house officer
Higher specialist training	Unified training grade
Continuing medical education	Consultant

and may be useful as a core syllabus on which didactic teaching or self-directed learning could be based.

The depth of coverage is more difficult to specify. At the level of general professional training, a broad understanding of each topic would be desirable (particularly Sections 1, 2 and 5–12). The higher specialist trainee would need to build on this by developing in-depth knowledge of particular aspects of nutrition directly relevant to a chosen specialty. For example, a trainee in perinatal medicine would need particularly to build on Sections 3–6 and 14, whereas Sections 14 and 16 would be of relevance to training in paediatric gastroenterology. The extent of nutrition training required would be specified by criteria for accreditation in the chosen subspecialty.

Implementation of nutrition education

Role of the British Paediatric Association and the Royal College of Physicians

The Standing Committee on Postgraduate Medical and Dental Education (SCOPME) has reported on the implications of *The health of the nation* for postgraduate medical education, remarking that:

> Few doctors ... have the necessary skills to be health promoters and would benefit from training.[10]

SCOPME concludes that education in health promotion must become an integral part of postgraduate medical education. Nutrition could clearly form a major part of health promotion curricula. The BPA, as the body principally responsible for advising on the content of paediatric training, is in a position both to increase the nutritional content of curricula and to set professional standards.

Examinations

Inclusion of nutrition topics in examinations is a powerful motivation to learn. Ensuring that nutrition comprises a fixed proportion of the questions in both undergraduate final examinations in child health and the MRCP Part 1 examination helps to stimulate interest. During higher specialist training, nutrition could form the basis of a course leading to acquisition of an MSc degree. Alternatively, nutrition may form a study module in other courses; an example exists in the MMedSci course established for senior registrars and senior clinical medical officers in Leeds (Rudolf MCJ; personal communication). The availability of a common syllabus (see Appendix) helps in the design of such initiatives.

Purchasing power

National Health Service (NHS) purchasing authorities could influence the priority accorded nutrition by specifying nutritional targets in contracts. The responsibilities of provider units and purchasing authorities in this area have been clearly set out in a recent DoH publication, *Nutrition and health: a management handbook for the NHS.*[11] Postgraduate deans, as purchasers of postgraduate medical education, also have power to influence this process. Greater emphasis on the purchasing of paediatric clinical nutrition as a service and educational resource is essential to the creation of specialist consultant posts in this area.

Conclusion

Improvements in the nutritional education of paediatricians in training have the potential to yield benefits in both the prevention and treatment of childhood disease. Obstacles to the achievement of this goal include the diffuse nature of nutrition and the failure to recognise clinical nutrition as a subspecialty in paediatrics. If these problems are to be overcome, a nutrition syllabus needs to be integrated vertically and horizontally into the curricula of undergraduates and paediatricians in training. NHS purchasing authorities, provider units, undergraduate and postgraduate deans, and examining bodies could all help to implement necessary changes in attitude to clinical nutrition.

References

1. King's Fund Centre. *A positive approach to nutrition as treatment.* London: King's Fund Centre, 1992
2. Poskitt EME, Williams AF, Jackson AA. A core paediatric nutrition curriculum for medical students. *Postgraduate Medical Journal* 1993; **69** (Suppl 2): S62
3. Department of Health. *The health of the nation—a strategy for health in England.* London: HMSO, 1992
4. Nutrition Task Force Project Team on Nutrition Education and Training for Health Professionals. *Core curriculum for nutrition in the education of health professionals.* London: HMSO, 1994
5. Southgate DAT (editorial). Images of nutrition. *British Journal of Nutrition* 1992; **67**: 147–8
6. National Institute of Child Health and Human Development. Five-year plan for nutrition research and training: executive summary. *Pediatric Research* 1992; **32**: 1–9

7. McLaren DS. Nutrition in medical schools: a case of mistaken identity. *American Journal of Clinical Nutrition* 1994; **59**: 960–3

8. Department of Health, Committee on Medical Aspects of Food Policy. *Dietary reference values for food energy and nutrients for the United Kingdom.* Reports on Health and Social Subjects 41. London: HMSO, 1991

9. Standing Committee on Nutrition, British Paediatric Association. *Core programme for the teaching and training of paediatric nutrition.* London: BPA, 1993

10. Standing Committee on Postgraduate Medical and Dental Education. *The health of the nation: the implications for postgraduate and continuing medical and dental education.* London: SCOPME, 1994

11. Nutrition Task Force. *Nutrition and health: a management handbook for the NHS.* London: Department of Health, 1994

APPENDIX: Core nutrition curriculum for paediatricians in training

1 *Growth*

   Measurement of growth; anthropometry

   Growth charts and interpretation

   Growth and nutrient accretion; reference fetus and infant

   Measurement of body composition

2 *Estimating nutrient requirements*

   Population approach; reference nutrient intake, lower reference nutrient intake, estimated average requirement

   Experimental approach; factorial method, nutrient balances, calorimetry

   Nutrient turnover; measurement and relevance; obligatory nutrient losses

   Methods of dietary assessment

3 *Nutrition in pregnancy*

   Periconceptional nutrition

   Nutrient requirements during pregnancy

   Malnutrition and effects on fetus

   Fetal growth disorders and significance

   Critical growth periods

4 *Low birth weight infant*

   Nutritional reserve

   Physiological limitations; protein quality and essential amino acids, solute load, acid-base balance, gastrointestinal adaptation

Fat absorption; essential fatty acids

Glucose turnover and homoeostasis

Energy balance; protein-energy interaction

Bone growth and mineralisation

Specific macro- and micro-nutrient requirements

5 *Lactation*

Regulation of milk production

Factors influencing nutritional composition; breast milk nitrogen

'Non-nutritional' aspects; host-defence, growth factors and adaptation

Morbidity associated with artificial feeding

Epidemiology of infant feeding

Maternal nutrition and lactation

Initiation of breast feeding

Mechanics of breast feeding and pathology

Common problems and practical management

Drugs and breast milk

6 *Breast milk substitutes*

Rationale for composition

Modification of cow's milk

Types of, and indications for, special milks

World Health Organisation code on marketing of breast milk substitutes

7 *Weaning and dietary supplements in infancy*

Definition; nutritional and other functions of weaning

Appropriate timing of weaning and justification

The weaning process; appropriate and inappropriate foods

Iron deficiency

Vitamin supplements (particularly vitamins D and K)

Requirements of babies born pre-term

Weaning problems: vegetarian baby, ethnic aspects, allergy and food intolerance in infancy

Failure-to-thrive (nutritional aspects)

8 *Pre-school child*
   Behavioural eating disorders: management and prevention
   The child with neurological disability

9 *The school child and adolescent*
   Diet of schoolchildren and potential for nutritional deficiency
   Vegetarianism and ethnic nutrition
   Anorexia and bulimia

10 *Obesity*
    Predisposing factors; epidemiology
    Outcome
    Management
    Long-term consequences

11 *Dental health and diet*
    Sugars
    Fluoride

12 *Sociological influences and nutrition policy*
    The health of the nation dietary targets
    Sociological influences and behaviour among various age groups
    Nutrition education; methods of changing behaviour and their
    efficacy

13 *International child health and nutrition*
    Nutritional assessment
    Influence of malnutrition on disease susceptibility
    Protein-energy malnutrition
    Vitamin deficiencies
    Nutritional rehabilitation

14 *Nutrition support*
    Indications
    Choice of enteral or parenteral route
    Devices: enteral and parenteral
    Devising parenteral nutrition regimens
    Types of enteral feed: polymeric, elemental and specialised

Objectives of nutrition support in gastrointestinal disease, oncology, renal disease, cardiopulmonary disease, traumatised surgical patients, acute and chronic neurological disability

15 *Nutritional management of metabolic disorders*
Amino acid requirements
Urea metabolism and disorders
Vitamin dependency
Hyperlipidaemias
Diabetes mellitus

16 *Food allergy and food intolerance*
Distinction between allergy and intolerance of various types
Food and systemic allergic disease (asthma, eczema)
Coeliac disease and gastrointestinal food intolerance

18 Nutritional problems in less developed countries

Andrew Tomkins
Director, Centre for International Child Health, Institute of Child Health
(University of London)

Children in less developed countries have a range of nutritional problems. The most visible is protein-energy malnutrition, but deficiencies of vitamin A, iodine and iron are also important as is the range of clinical syndromes associated with mineral and trace element deficiencies. Nutritional excesses occur in several situations. The increasing prevalence of obesity, due to inappropriate diet, and of fluorosis, due to environmental problems, are just two examples.

Nomenclature

The term 'malnutrition' is often used for children whose weight or height departs significantly from international growth standards, and 'severe malnutrition' usually for the severe, clinically recognisable syndromes of kwashiorkor, marasmus and marasmic kwashiorkor. The basic causes of malnutrition include poverty, lack of availability of food, infection and inadequate care. National nutritional policies usually focus on production and requirement for energy and protein intakes, perhaps neglecting the micronutrient and mineral deficiencies that may occur in the presence of relatively satisfactory protein and energy status. Similarly, the term 'household food security', increasingly used to describe the ability of families to grow and/or purchase enough food for all family members, tends to focus on energy and protein alone. It is perhaps therefore preferable to use the term malnutrition in a generic way to include a range of nutritional deficiencies, and then specify the nature, severity and functional disability associated with that particular deficiency.

Many conceptual models describe the basis of malnutrition as poverty together with poor household food security, both of which are determined by economics, politics, international and national relationships, climate and agricultural resources. However, these general factors are considerably influenced by the presence of infection (Figure 1). The overall outcome of nutritional deficiency may be detected as disordered function of cells, tissues or entire organs.[1] This is most strikingly seen in the impact of malnutrition syndromes on the immune system rendering children more susceptible to severe infections and increasing their risk of dying from specific infections.[2] Case fatality rates for several childhood infections vary considerably between different communities, much of the difference being accounted for by variation in the severity of nutritional deficiency.[3]

In seeking to improve nutritional status there are several approaches, each with its own terminology:

- *dietary diversification*: improved range and quantity of intake of food items;
- *fortification*: the enrichment of food such as salt or sugar with elements such as iron or iodine;
- *supplementation*: specific doses such as capsules of solutions containing vitamin A or D given with prophylactic or therapeutic regimens.

Infection/nutrition relationships

It is now well recognised that several childhood infections have a profound influence on nutritional status. These include persistent diarrhoea, measles, HIV, pertussis, tuberculosis and malaria. Con-

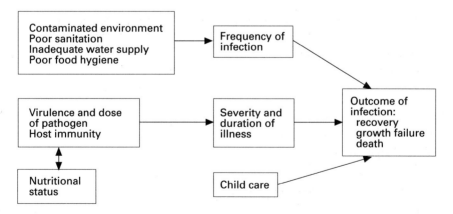

Fig. 1. *Diagrammatic representation of the relationship between infection and nutritional status and of the mechanisms of nutritional change during infection.*

siderable attention has been given to the interface between nutrition and diarrhoeal disease. A study of dietary intake and intestinal loss of energy during episodes of persistent diarrhoea among Gambian children[4] showed a striking reduction in dietary energy intake during the illness (to about 60 kcal per kg body weight per day) but, despite quite marked persistent diarrhoea, only 10% of dietary energy was lost in the faeces. During the convalescent period, dietary intake increased to about 135 kcal per kg body weight per day, again with a 5–10% intestinal loss of energy.

Recent studies have emphasised the variety of reasons why nutritional status may deteriorate during illness (Table 1):

- there may be strong cultural beliefs among the carers, with certain foods avoided and others given in more dilute concentrations;
- there may be quite marked biochemical control of the appetite— several recent studies have emphasised the importance of cytokines which are released in infection and cause an inhibition of the appetite centre;
- appetite is frequently decreased in episodes of pyrexia, possibly due to the increased circulating cytokine levels;
- buccal lesions such as *Monilia* infection may frequently complicate diarrhoeal disease and make eating painful;
- similarly, abdominal pain and the anal discomfort of persistent diarrhoea contribute to the general misery and reduced dietary intake;

Table 1. Some of the mechanisms whereby infections cause malnutrition

- Withholding of certain foods
- Production of cytokines
- Anorexia
- Pyrexia
- Increase in nutrient requirements
- Catabolic losses
- Malabsorption
- Production of acute-phase proteins
- Decreased serum levels of micronutrients
- Impairment of immune response

- experimental, and some clinical, studies suggest that zinc deficiency, frequently present among children with moderate or severe protein-energy malnutrition, may lead to anorexia;[5] and
- experimental studies suggest that potassium deficiency may also cause anorexia.

Repletion of these deficiencies during diarrhoeal management is crucial for the achievement of satisfactory weight gain.[6]

Household food technology to increase dietary intake

Amylase-rich flour

Several recent studies have examined the impact of decreasing viscosity of weaning foods by the use of amylase-rich flour. Amylase hydrolyses starch and therefore decreases the viscosity, enabling additional quantities of dry matter to be added during the preparation of the weaning food, producing an isoviscous consistency with increased energy and protein content. The reduction of a thick gruel to a thin liquid with the consistency of soup is striking. In a recent study in Tanzania, the use of amylase-rich flour resulted in a 40% increase in dietary energy intake among children admitted to a paediatric ward with severe diarrhoea.[7] Amylase can be produced locally using a simple sprouting technique with millet, sorghum, maize or rice. It is found in greatest concentration in the shoots; once the grains have sprouted, the shoots may be ground to make an amylase-rich flour which, when added in a concentration of 1 in 100, produces a striking reduction in viscosity.

Fermentation of cereals

Many communities ferment cereals before cooking. This has several advantages:[8]
- the pH is reduced to about 3.6, which is markedly inhibitory to many micro-organisms;
- antibiotics are produced during the fermentation process; and
- the improved taste of the fermented food often acts as a stimulant to appetite during illness.

The protective effect of fermented foods taken regularly in children's diets against their susceptibility to diarrhoea has been investigated in Tanzania recently. Children in villages regularly consuming fermented food had significantly less diarrhoea than those in villages taking non-fermented cereals.[9]

Impact of deworming on nutrition

Many children in less developed countries are infected with a range of geohelminths, such as *Ascaris, Trichuris, Schistosoma* (*haematobium* and *mansoni*) and *Strongyloides*. They may also be infected with hookworm, amoeba and *Giardia*. The impact of these parasites on nutritional status varies according to the load of parasite and the underlying nutritional status, but there may be considerable benefits of deworming on growth, iron status, vitamin A, zinc, cognitive function, school achievement and physical fitness. The availability of single-dose drugs such as albendazole now makes it possible for children to be dewormed on a regular basis, say at the beginning of each academic term, using relatively low cost drugs. The therapeutic impact of albendazole or mebendazole and praziquantel should be combined with intensive efforts on health education to prevent re-infection.[10] Unfortunately, despite considerable environmental gains due to improved sanitation and water supplies, the nutrition of millions of children is still compromised by intestinal parasites.[11] Health education programmes in schools should be promoted strongly, but they may have a limited effect unless they are combined with better environmental control and chemotherapy.

Specific deficiencies

Vitamin A deficiency and infection

It has been known for many decades that severe vitamin A deficiency is associated with increased susceptibility to infection and mortality but the impact of mild or moderate subclinical deficiency has been unclear. About 10 major studies have been performed during the last decade in which vitamin A intake was improved by dietary approaches using regular daily supplements of small doses of vitamin A, by fortification of food items or by large doses of vitamin A administered every four months. Overall, there was a remarkably consistent reduction in mortality whichever method was used, with about 20% decrease in mortality among children below 60 months of age in those areas where vitamin A deficiency was proven to be present. Considering the many millions of children who live in such areas, the impact on infant and child mortality of widespread prophylaxis could be considerable.

A recent study in Ghana (Ghana VAST) showed, like several others, a 20% reduction in mortality, but it also explored the different types of illness which contributed to the overall mortality in the placebo and intervention groups.[12] There was an overall decrease in the number of clinic attendances and hospital admissions. The mortality from acute diarrhoeal disease was significantly reduced by four-monthly administration of vitamin A, and there was a trend towards reduction in mortality among children with persistent diarrhoea and malnutrition. Interestingly, there was no significant impact of vitamin A on deaths from measles in this study, which contrasts with studies of children with such severe measles that they required hospital admission in which there was a significant reduction in mortality if the children were given large doses of vitamin A soon after admission.

Recent studies have examined the impact of infection on vitamin A levels in the blood, noting that the presence of malaria parasites, even in asymptomatic children, is an important cause of low levels of vitamin A. The difference between zero parasites and a heavy parasitaemia accounted for a 30% reduction in plasma vitamin A.[13] In addition, when some of the acute-phase proteins were measured in the blood of children in the Ghana VAST study there was a striking increase in C-reactive protein and alpha-1 acid glycoprotein in the vitamin A supplemented children compared with the placebo group. It appears therefore that the acute-phase response is stimulated by vitamin A supplementation and this may in some way be protective against severe diarrhoea. It is interesting that vitamin A did not affect the acute-phase response in other illnesses. This raises the intriguing possibility that vitamin A supplementation produces a different anti-inflammatory effect according to the site of the infection.

A recent study from Malawi emphasises the impressive association between vitamin A deficiency and perinatal transmission of HIV from mother to infant.[14] Furthermore, mothers with vitamin A deficiency were more likely to experience death of their infants than women with better vitamin A levels. Although this study controlled for a number of variables, it is still possible that vitamin A deficiency is a marker of other deficiencies, both in diet and in access to health services. There are, however, many biologically plausible reasons why vitamin A might influence the perinatal transmission of HIV:

- the impact of vitamin A on epithelial cell structure and mucus production could influence the entry of HIV through reproductive tract epithelium and may increase susceptibility to sexually transmitted diseases;

- abnormal epithelial structure might also increase susceptibility to HIV transmission during the birth process; and

- vitamin A deficiency could also increase the risk of transmission of HIV through breast milk by altering immune responses.

Whatever the biological plausibility, ultimately the only way of knowing whether vitamin A is so important a risk for perinatal transmission of HIV is to perform intervention studies at different stages of pregnancy.

Zinc deficiency

The association between zinc deficiency and shortness of stature, impaired linear growth, decreased immune function and susceptibility to disease has been recognised for several decades. More recently, zinc deficiency has been demonstrated in moderate and severe protein-energy malnutrition.[5] Addition of zinc acetate to standard nutrition rehabilitation regimens of dried skimmed milk, sugar and oil, or cereal/pulse mixes, has been accompanied by an improved rate of catch-up growth and improvement in the immune function.[5] Zinc has profound effects on the intestinal epithelium in experimental studies where there is atrophy of the intestinal mucosa and the development of diarrhoea. When cholera toxin is perfused in such situations there is a heightened secretion of water and electrolytes.

With this information in mind, studies were established in Bangladesh to investigate the impact of zinc acetate supplementation in children with acute or persistent diarrhoea who also had moderate or severe protein-energy malnutrition.[15] The addition of zinc acetate did not influence the loss of fluid in stools or the duration of diarrhoea in children with mild protein-energy malnutrition but there was significant decrease in stool volume in those moderately or severely malnourished, and a significant shortening of the duration of symptoms among such children with persistent diarrhoea. Furthermore, the number of episodes of diarrhoea during the three-month follow-up period after discharge was significantly reduced by a two-week course of zinc acetate. These effects appear quite striking but there is a strong possibility that combinations of minerals and micronutrients might produce an even more beneficial effect, and studies are underway. These studies have practical implications for feeding regimens among refugee populations, and minerals/micronutrient mixes are now commercially available for addition to cereal/pulse mixes in camps.

Iodine deficiency disorders

Iodine deficiency can cause a range of clinical syndromes from cretinism at its most severe to moderate disorders of impaired cognitive function and neuromuscular coordination in milder deficiency[16]—indeed, it is the commonest cause of disability globally. Typically, iodine deficiency has been associated with volcanic rock and mountains where the iodine content of soil has been shown to be particularly low. However, it is increasingly recognised that iodine is eluted from the soil by repeated flooding. Thus, subjects with iodine deficiency disorder may live in mountainous regions such as the Himalayas and also in flat terrains such as in the riverine areas in Bangladesh.[17] The most crucial period is pregnancy: if the mother is unable to take enough iodine she becomes hypothyroid, with potentially devastating effects on the development of the infant's brain *in utero*.

Salt iodisation has been demonstrated to be effective but there are considerable logistic problems for many communities in less developed countries:

1. There may be no legislation and therefore no stimulation to provide iodised salt. This is a particular problem in countries that import their salt from other countries.

2. There may be no commercial equipment suitable for iodising salt. Although the iodine spraying equipment is relatively simple, it requires maintenance and good quality control.

3. There may be problems of distributing the iodised salt to the communities, particularly those in remote mountainous areas.

4. If the salt is left unattended in the open, it is all too easily soaked by rain and the iodine leached out.

Thus, alternative approaches have been put forward. The most popular until recently was a single injectable source of iodine given as lipiodol which is considered to protect the pregnant woman for 3–5 years. However, with the increasing concern about the high prevalence of hepatitis B and HIV, there are problems with this approach. Similarly, it is expensive in terms of labour because of the need for trained nursing staff.

An alternative, simpler approach has been developed in the last decade. This consists of a capsule of iodised poppy seed oil which can be given as a single oral dose which may be effective for 2–3 years. A single dose given in early pregnancy may protect against effects on the infant *in utero*, but it is not yet clear whether similar results will be obtained in malnourished subjects with deficiency of body fat (where much of the iodised oil is stored) and different levels of intensity of intestinal parasitic infection.

Setting targets for nutrition and monitoring activities

At the Summit for Children in 1992, the majority of the world's governments signed a commitment towards action on at least six major activities. These included reduction in the prevalence of low birth weight, elimination of vitamin A and iodine deficiency, reduction in protein-energy malnutrition and iron deficiency, and support of exclusive breast feeding.[18]

Birth weight

Low birth weight can be due to intra-uterine growth retardation and/or premature delivery. In less developed countries the majority of low birth weight infants (less than 2.5 kg) are due to the former. A range of maternal and infant risk factors may be identified which differ in their relative strengths from community to community throughout the world. Assessing the prevalence of low birth weight is difficult enough in hospitals where scales may not be accurate or attention to detail unsatisfactory, but it is even more difficult in the community because of a lack of scales that can be used in the home. Simple spring scales are available for weighing children less than 2.5 kg, but their sensitivity and specificity in relation to more accurate scales have yet to be determined. Several approaches such as tapes for measurement of skull circumference (a good indicator of body weight) may be useful in the future. The percentage of infants with low birth weight ranges from less than 7% in the more industrialised countries to over 50% in poorer countries such as rural Bangladesh. Improving birth weight will require major integrated approaches emphasising improvements in diet, toxic exposure, management of infection and physical activity.

Vitamin A

Surveys of vitamin A deficiency used to rely on ocular manifestations using the World Health Organisation (WHO) criteria for grades of xerophthalmia. However, even in the most severely affected areas less than 1% of children have night blindness, and it is generally agreed that eye surveys are labour expensive, usually requiring about 6,000 subjects to be examined by trained ocular health professionals. More recently, investigators have assessed the value of conjunctival impression cytology in which mucus secretion, which is decreased in vitamin A deficiency, is examined microscopically in conjunctival impression smears. Unfortunately, the sensitivity and specificity of this test have been rather unsatisfactory. Most surveys now measure plasma retinol, but the interpretation of a single level of plasma retinol requires caution because of the impact of infection.[13] Several newer methods using the relative and the modified relative dose responses have been introduced, but even these appear to be affected by infection. At present, therefore, it seems that the population distribution of plasma retinol, taken at a single time point, may well be the best indicator for progress. Each country will have to develop its own strategy for elimination of vitamin A deficiency; this will mostly involve a combination of dietary diversification, fortification and supplementation.

Iodine

Programmes of iodisation of salt have been made considerably easier by simple portable kits whereby trained field-workers can assess the iodine content of salt using a simple starch test. The impact of iodisation on humans can be assessed by measurement of the percentage with abnormal levels of thyroid-stimulating hormone (TSH) and thyroxine (T4), both of which can be measured on small blood samples on filter paper. In certain conditions, iodisation of the salt may need to be given in larger quantities because of existing goitrogens and selenium deficiency. However, there does not appear to be any iodine-deficient community whose thyroid function cannot be normalised by the administration of large amounts of iodine.

Protein energy malnutrition

The proportion of children who are malnourished with respect to weight, height and mid-upper arm circumference may be assessed by community studies using the basic EPI (expanded programme of immunisation) cluster sampling programme in which 30 clusters, each containing seven subjects, are measured. Cut-off values of less than 2Z scores, for weight for age, height for age, or weight for height, may be used and may be accompanied by measurements of thinness. The mid-upper arm circumference is associated with increased mortality below a value of 12.5 and sharper increase below 11.5 and 10.5; these cut-offs have been used in a variety of surveys.[3] Similarly, the body mass index (weight divided by height squared) has been used among school-age children.

Iron

The Summit for Children emphasised a reduction in iron deficiency in keeping with the functional deficits associated with iron deficiency.[19] One of the problems facing those wishing to assess iron deficiency in less developed countries is the striking impact of systemic infection on 'iron indicators'. Serum iron, total iron binding capacity and ferritin are all increased by systemic infection, which may lead to underestimation of the level of iron deficiency in a community. The introduction of newer indices for iron status such as the transferrin receptor assays needs further evaluation but these may well be less susceptible to modulation from the acute-phase response. In the meantime, haemoglobin, as an index of iron status, is likely to remain popular and widely used.

Breast feeding

The importance of the support of exclusive breast feeding for the first four months of life cannot be overemphasised. In practice, there seem to be many sources of advice and advertising that persuade women against exclusive breast feeding despite the clear guidelines of the WHO code.

Challenges for the future

The Cairo conference on population in 1994 emphasised the problems for nutrition of children associated with the marked increase in population in some countries. The reasons for population increase are complex, but overall the message from surveys among women in less developed countries is that family planning services are often inadequate, unattractive, inefficient and lacking in confidentiality. It is no longer reasonable to say that certain communities *always* wish to have large families for cultural reasons.

Infant and young child mortality and malnutrition rates have fallen in nearly all countries over the last two decades,[18] but there is now a disturbing slowing of rates of improvement, and in some countries a reversal. Wars and civil disturbances precipitate serious nutritional problems in countries which are only marginally food secure. Health and nutrition services for children must use appropriate technology which is not only biologically successful and culturally attractive but also affordable and available, within either a government health system or some form of private, parallel drug distribution or sale system. There is an increasing need for doctors and nurses to play an advocacy role in the changing climate of health care and nutrition provision. Health sector reforms and market forces may improve 'efficiency' but decrease 'availability' of health and nutrition services for vulnerable groups of children.

Agencies such as the World Bank have identified nutrition as a good investment. Whether the development of adequate nutrition is regarded as a basic human right or as essential building blocks in the development of healthy individuals, improvement of nutrition status can be sustained only by the combined activities of health professionals and their colleagues in the related departments of agriculture, economics, education and social welfare. Too much energy is put into single sector approaches. The challenge for the future is to develop clearly defined health and nutrition pro-grammes, with specific preventive and therapeutic inputs by several cadres of workers, with doctors, nurses and nutritionists playing a major role.

References

1. Tomkins AM, Watson F. *Malnutrition and infection: a review.* Advisory Committee on Coordination/Subcommittee on Nutrition. Nutrition policy discussion paper no. 5 Geneva: World Health Organisation, 1989: 1–136
2. Chandra RK. Increased bacterial binding to respiratory epithelial cells in vitamin A deficiency. *British Medical Journal* 1988; **297**: 834–5
3. Vella V, Tomkins AM, Ndiku J, Marshal T, Cortinovis I. Anthropometry as a predictor for mortality among Ugandan children allowing for socio-economic variables. *European Journal of Clinical Nutrition* 1994; **48**: 189–97
4. Tomkins AM. Nutritional cost of protracted diarrhoea in young Gambian children. *Gut* 1983; **24**: A495
5. Golden MHN, Golden BE. Plasma zinc, rate of weight gain and the energy cost of tissue deposition in children recovering from severe malnutrition on a cow's milk or soya protein based diet. *American Journal of Clinical Nutrition* 1981; **34**: 892–9
6. Waterlow JC. *Protein energy malnutrition.* London, New York: Edward Arnold, 1992: 1–404
7. Darling JC, Kitundu JA, Kingamkono RP, Msengi AE, *et al.* Improved energy intakes using amylase-digested weaning foods in Tanzanian children with acute diarrhoea. *Journal of Pediatric Gastroenterology and Nutrition* 1995 (in press)
8. Mensah P, Tomkins AM, Drasar BS, Harrison TJ. Fermentation of cereals for reduction of bacterial contamination of weaning foods in Ghana. *Lancet* 1990; **336**: 140–3
9. Lorri W, Svanberg U. Lower prevalence of diarrhoea in young children fed lactic acid-fermented gruels. *Food and Nutrition Bulletin* 1994; **15**(1): 57–63
10. Savioli L, Bundy D, Tomkins AM. Intestinal parasitic infections: a soluble public health problem. *Transactions of the Royal Society of Tropical Medicine and Hygiene* 1992; **86**: 353–4
11. Stephenson LS. *The impact of helminth infections on human nutrition.* London, New York, Philadelphia: Taylor and Francis, 1987: 1–223

12. Ghana VAST Study Team. Vitamin A supplementation in northern Ghana: effects on clinic attendances, hospital admissions, and child mortality. *Lancet* 1993; **342**: 7–12

13. Filteau SM, Morris SS, Abbott RA, Tomkins AM, *et al.* Influence of morbidity on serum retinol of children in a community-based study in northern Ghana. *American Journal of Clinical Nutrition* 1993; **58**: 192–7

14. Semba RD, Miotti PG, Chiphangwi JD, Saah AJ, *et al.* Maternal vitamin A deficiency and mother-to-child transmission of HIV-1. *Lancet* 1994; **343**: 1593–7

15. Roy SK, Behrens RH, Haider R, Akramuzzaman SM, *et al.* Impact of zinc supplementation on intestinal permeability in Bangladeshi children with acute diarrhoea and persistent diarrhoea syndrome. *Journal of Pediatric Gastroenterology and Nutrition* 1992; **15**: 289–96

16. Hetzel BS. *The story of iodine deficiency: an international challenge in nutrition.* Oxford, New York, Tokyo: Oxford University Press, 1989: 1–236

17. Filteau SM, Sullivan KR, Anwar US, Anwar ZR, Tomkins AM. Iodine deficiency alone cannot account for goitre prevalence among pregnant women in Modhupur, Bangladesh. *European Journal of Clinical Nutrition* 1994; **48**: 293–302

18. Grant JP. The state of the world's children. UNICEF, Oxford University Press, 1993: 1–90

19. Bates CJ, Evans PH, Allison G. Biochemical indices and neuromuscular function tests in rural Gambian schoolchildren given a riboflavin, or multivitamin plus iron, supplement. *British Journal of Nutrition* 1994; **72**: 601–10

19 | The Health of the Nation: the population perspective

Alan A Jackson
Professor of Human Nutrition and Director, Institute of Human Nutrition, University of Southampton School of Biological Sciences; Honorary Consultant in Clinical Nutrition, Southampton University Hospitals Trust

The last 10–15 years have seen a remarkable change in the perception of nutritional issues of public health importance. There has been substantial progress in the general move towards concerns of direct relevance to public health and their promotion as important issues within the national arena. Almost invariably the issues are complex, and therefore contentious, and impact importantly upon the economic well-being of one or other aspect of the food industry in general.

The early period of the 1980s was marked by two reports, neither of which was accepted by the commissioning agency but both of which served to mould the thoughts and approaches developed over the succeeding decade. The Black report on inequalities in health was not formally accepted in 1980;[1,2] the National Advisory Committee on Nutrition Education report on proposals for nutritional guidelines for health education was treated in a similar way in 1983.[3] Together, and also in their individual ways, both documents had a powerful determinant influence on perceptions of the need for change in wide sectors of society. The shift in emphasis took time to develop, and required a more formal marshalling of the scientific evidence to support and justify the positions adopted in the reports.

The most eloquent expression of the shift in emphasis is illustrated by the government's adoption of the White Paper *The Health of the Nation* in 1993.[4] The stated objective of the proposals within the White Paper was to 'add years to life and life to years'. Five key areas were identified for immediate action:

- cardiovascular disease;
- cancer;
- accidents;
- mental health; and
- HIV.

On the surface, none of these appeared to be explicitly related to nutrition, but in fact most carried either direct or indirect implications for nutrition, with identified targets within the key area of cardiovascular disease. The need to coordinate the wide range of activities of direct relevance to nutrition and changing the dietary intake of the nation led to the formation of the National Task Force on Nutrition which has articulated its goals and plans for actions in *Eat well*.[5] In Scotland the approach has been more direct, with the formulation of a 'national diet'.[6] This remarkable shift in emphasis owes a great deal to the persistence of pressure groups and to the quality of the scientific enquiry—often guided by individuals originally trained in public health nutrition for the developing world.

In the paediatric context, public health places emphasis on normal growth and development and the promotion of well-being rather than on the identification, treatment and management of recognised disease conditions. The overall objectives are different from those for adults. For childhood, the goal in biological terms is growth, development and ordered maturation to reach reproductive competency; in social terms, it is a well rounded, socially competent and productive member of society. Although longevity is clearly important, it cannot be sought at the expense of the other objectives.

There are two issues in childhood health for which the evidence is clear and immediate action is justified:

- supplementation with folic acid to prevent neural tube defects; and

- breast feeding to promote well-being and prevent diarrhoeal disease and respiratory infections during the first three months of life.

There are other issues of great importance for which there is the need to develop clear and unambiguous policies, one of the most important being the nutritional health of adolescents, especially in the context of teenage pregnancy.

Folic acid and neural tube defects

The government responded rapidly to the findings of the Medical Research Council prospective study on the effect of folic acid supplementation during pregnancy on neural tube defects.[7] An expert committee was convened under the chairmanship of Dame June Lloyd, and its deliberations were reported and published within the year.[8] The appropriate response in public health terms is still awaited for a condition which makes excessive demands on paediatric time in terms of the care and emotional support of the victims and their families.

After a five-year study, Wald and his colleagues showed conclusively that supplementation with 4 mg/day of folic acid during the periconceptional period reduced by 70% the risk of a recurrence of neural tube defect in women at risk.[7] (In fact, only a minority of defects are recurrences, with 90% being first occurrences.) The Chief Medical Officer (CMO) issued the following advice:

- women at high risk of having a child with a neural tube defect should receive supplemental folic acid, 4 mg/day, from the time they consider getting pregnant until the 12th week of pregnancy;
- to prevent an occurrence, all women at risk of becoming pregnant should take *additional* folic acid, 400 µg/day, until the 12th week of pregnancy.[8]

As the reference nutrient intake for folic acid is 200 µg per day, this means a total daily intake of 600 µg. Although it is theoretically possible to obtain this amount of folate in the diet, it is unlikely that most women will achieve it, even with a special effort. For this reason, it was further recommended that supplemental folic acid be taken by all women in the reproductive years.

This advice has been widely circulated through formal channels, but its implications have still not attracted the level of attention needed for effective implementation.

Breast feeding, diarrhoeal disease and respiratory infection

It was a surprise to many people that breast feeding and its promotion were not identified within the targets of *The Health of the Nation*. There are undoubtedly several reasons for this, and its omission should not lead to the mistaken perception that breast feeding has been either forgotten or ignored. Indeed, to provide a specific focus on breast feeding, a national breast feeding working group was established in December 1992. It currently has three primary objectives:

- to develop educational resources;
- to heighten public awareness; and
- to offer guidance to health authorities.

Surveys to determine the pattern of breast feeding have been carried out every five years since 1980, and a breast feeding promotion campaign has been in operation since 1988. The surveys show little change in either the frequency or the pattern of breast feeding across the UK over the past decade. There is a marked age and social class divide in the prevalence of breast feeding, with lowest rates in the youngest mothers and the lowest social groups.[9]

The classic study reported by Howie and colleagues from Dundee[10] makes it incontrovertibly clear that the risk of respiratory or gastrointestinal disease during early life is increased 5–15 fold in infants who are not breast fed but given an artificial formulation. Based upon this evidence, there can be no argument that the single most important factor to reduce the burden of ill health during the first year of life in this country at the present time is to ensure that as many infants as possible are breast fed for the first three months of life. This has to be one of the most important responsibilities of a paediatrician. Given the high rate of potentially life-threatening complications associated with artificial formulations, they should be viewed as therapeutic interventions for management as a last resort.

Nutrition in adolescence

All health messages directed at mothers should take into account the fact that many first-time mothers are teenagers themselves and still adolescents. Adolescents are a complex group with whom to deal, an age group in transition from one state to another. Nevertheless, they represent the end-product of the paediatrician's attention and, as parents, the start of the next cycle of concern.

During adolescence, the variable timing and responsiveness of the growth spurt and the attendant biological changes (hormonal, physical and sexual) produce complex patterns of emotional responses and social maturation. The emotional problems associated with moving from dependency to independence carry their own inherent risks. During a period in which there are special risks for health, the fact that this age group is poorly catered for in health terms, tending to fall between two sets of caring, only adds to the difficulties.

In his report, *On the state of public health, 1993,* the CMO highlights the special problems and needs of this particular group.[11] In terms of public health, many of the problems are directly related to issues of lifestyle. Although smoking is declining in most population groups, it is not declining among teenagers.[12] Smokers tend to take a diet which is intrinsically less healthy, so this pattern of behaviour has direct nutritional implications.[13] Alcohol, drug abuse and sexual activity all carry attendant risks. The use of special diets for such reasons as concerns about body image or health has led to an increase in non-traditional dietary patterns (eg vegetarianism),[14] and a marked increase in the frequency of pathological eating disorders (eg the anorexia-related syndromes).[15] Patterns of physical activity start to be set in adolescence which are likely to determine lifelong behaviour. All this is happening at the same time as young people are preparing themselves to be parents for the first time, and to begin to accept responsibility for the well-being of the next generation.

Dietary patterns in adolescence

We are fortunate in the UK to have nationally representative data collected on a regular basis on food supplies, diet and health. Although adolescents have never been identified as a discrete group for these surveys, a separate analysis was made for the age group 16–24 in the *Dietary and nutritional survey of British adults* in 1986–87,[16] and an increasing number of studies have looked at aspects of the diets of adolescents in England,[17,18] Scotland,[19] and Northern Ireland.[20]

It is no surprise, but sobering to note, that in the national survey the diet of the 16–24 age group was characterised as consisting of convenience foods, snacks and confectionery, with a notable shortage of fresh fruit and vegetables. In nutritional terms, this translates to concern about the adequacy of specific nutrients, especially calcium, vitamins A and D, iron and riboflavin.[16] This general pattern is reflected in other surveys and smaller studies.

Rugg-Gunn's group carried out a detailed dietary survey in 11–12 year olds in Newcastle in 1980.[21] In 1990, using similar methodologies, they studied the nutrient intake and status of 379 children aged 11–12 years—thus enabling a direct comparison between 1980 and 1990.[17] In general, the children in 1990 were taller and heavier than in 1980. As body mass index has also increased, they were heavier for their height than a decade ago. Therefore, they have grown *more*, but it is an open question whether they have grown *better*. This increase in size has occurred despite an overall reduction in total energy intake, strongly suggesting a decrease in the general physical activity in this population, reflecting the decreased levels of activity reported for schoolchildren in other studies.[22] Although the total energy intake was reduced in the later study, this was not reflected in a similar level of reduction of many nutrients, implying that the diet had become more nutrient-dense. There was a social class gradient for this change, with the nutrient density increase being most evident in the higher social classes, who also had the greatest reduction in total energy intake. There were no changes in sugar intake, and fat consistently provided about 40% of total energy, indicating little or no movement towards recommended dietary patterns.[17,23] About half of both the boys and the girls failed to achieve the population reference for calcium and iron intake.

Iron and calcium intake in adolescence

Concerns about the nutritional status for iron and calcium are based upon the demonstrated involvement of these nutrients in conditions of widespread public health concern. Iron deficiency has been shown to be directly related to physical growth and intellectual development, work capacity, mood and behaviour.[23] The evidence linking maternal iron deficiency anaemia to placental and fetal growth, in particular to an increase in the ratio of fetal weight to placental weight and the risk of hypertension in later life, makes it of considerable importance.[24]

Iron status and intake in adolescents has recently been investigated in some detail by Nelson and his colleagues.[14] In exploring the effect of ethnic background, they found that about 11% of white 11–14 year old girls in London were anaemic (haemoglobin <120 g/l) compared with 22% of Indian girls. The proportion of vegetarians amongst the Indians was twice that of the white girls, so it appeared at first sight that a vegetarian diet was a special risk factor for anaemia. However, when the data were examined in greater detail, being a vegetarian was found to be associated with a low haemoglobin only in the white girls; among the Indian girls the risk was greater for non-vegetarians. Lower haemoglobin levels were more common in girls who had tried to lose weight, in the families of manual workers, and those with earlier menarche. Physical performance was compromised in the girls with a low haemoglobin. Therefore, in this population the immediate causes of low haemoglobin represented a complex of factors related to their culture, lifestyle and personal biology. There is clearly a need for interventions at the personal and public health level, but the most appropriate approach requires careful consideration.

Osteoporosis and the risk of bone damage and fracture during later life are related directly to the achievement of peak bone mass; this is thought to be determined in large part by the dietary intake and availability of calcium during the period of growth.[23] With 40–50% of the skeletal mass deposited during adolescence, the impact of good dietary practice at this age may have important implications for musculoskeletal well-being in later life.

Valimiki *et al* have recently reported an opportunistic study in which they examined lifestyle factors associated with bone mineral density in the hip and vertebrae prospectively over 11 years in 264 adolescent males and females.[25] In the males, statistically significant associations were found with weight, exercise, age and smoking (negative), which together could explain 46% of the variance in bone density. In the females, significant associations were identified with weight, exercise and age, explaining 38% of the variance. When weight, exercise and age were not forced variables in the analysis there was an independent relationship between dietary calcium intake and bone density in the females. The reference intake for calcium in this age group in the UK is 800 mg/day. There was a statistically significant difference in bone density in those with an intake of calcium below or above 800 mg/day.[23] In the males, no relationship with calcium intake could be demonstrated, probably because they had an intake of 1,400 mg/day, which is above the threshold for the effect. The increased calcium intake in the males was attributed directly to milk consumption. The levels of activity used to differentiate the active and inactive groups were modest: two or more periods of activity of 30 minutes in a week compared with less than two periods.

The main sources of iron in the British diet are breakfast cereals, meat and meat products; for calcium, milk, bread and cheese; for vitamin D, dairy products and fortified yellow spreads (eg margarine).

At the present time in the UK, iron, calcium, niacin and thiamine are added to wheat flour to restore the levels removed by processing. Margarine is fortified by law with vitamin D and vitamin A to ensure that the levels are at least those found in butter.

The Department of Health published the *Dietary reference values for food energy and nutrients for the United Kingdom* in 1991.[23] This document represented an important and novel departure in a number of ways from previous reports dealing with recommendations on nutrient requirements for the population. One important difference was that, for the first time, dietary guidelines were explicitly developed within the document relating to:

- a reduction in the total fat content of the diet, particularly by reducing the amount of saturated fat; and

- changes in the pattern of carbohydrate consumption, with a decrease in simple sugars and an increase in complex carbohydrates such as starch and non-starch polysaccharides.

When translated into patterns of food intake, the guidelines emerge as the recommendations from the National Task Force on Nutrition, *The balance of good health.*[26]

Whilst fully supporting these proposals, it needs to be carefully considered how they can be applied effectively to adolescents as a critical subgroup, without running the risk of exposing them to nutrient imbalances of the kind discussed above. Clearly, this requires further judicious thought and consideration.

Activity: primary driver for healthy nutrition

To a great extent nutritional well-being represents the balance between energy expenditure and food intake. Within this relationship the beneficial role played by an increase in physical activity justifies considerable emphasis. It has a direct effect in generating a metabolic demand for iron and calcium. At the same time, the increased energy expenditure leads to an increase in food intake, and hence an increase in nutrient intake. The consequence is that an increase in activity enables an adequate intake even of nutrients which may be relatively low in the total diet. The wide range of other physiological and metabolic benefits, either directly caused by or associated with an increase in physical activity, is becoming increasingly more evident. The magnitude of the social class divide in physical activity is a cause for concern.

The future

At the present time, diet, nutrition and health enjoy a position on the national agenda of greater importance than at any time in the last 50 years. This is a direct consequence of the scientific enquiries which have demonstrated many direct links with health and have suggested an even wider range of potentially important interactions. In the past, public health interventions designed to address nutritional considerations directly have been effective but, by and large, have related to the eradication of deficiency disorders such as rickets and scurvy. Today the agenda is more complex: at the same time as consideration is given to deficiencies of folic acid, iron and calcium, reductions are being sought in the dietary components which have traditionally acted as the vehicle for some of these nutrients. The approaches to be adopted for dietary change and behaviour modification will have to draw on a wider range of professional skills than has been customary in the past.

It is reasonable to conclude that one of the most serious threats to public health is the well-being of adolescents, both in terms of their own risk as adults and the risk they convey to the next generation through parenting. The issues surrounding the dietary intake and requirements of adolescents are complex. Perhaps the single most important factor is the metabolic demand generated by activity to stimulate food intake. In this sense, the most important nutritional consideration in adolescence may be the level of habitual activity in which they engage.

References

1. Department of Health and Social Security. *Inequalities in health: report of a research working group.* London: Department of Health and Social Security, 1980
2. Townsend P, Davidson N. *Inequalities in health: the Black report.* Harmondsworth, Middlesex: Penguin Books, 1992
3. National Advisory Committee on Nutrition Education. *Discussion paper on proposals for nutritional guidelines for health education in Britain.* London: Health Education Council, 1983
4. Department of Health. *The Health of the Nation—a strategy for health in England.* London: HMSO, 1992
5. Nutrition Task Force. *Eat well.* An action plan to achieve *The health of the nation* targets on diet and nutrition. London: Department of Health, 1994
6. The Scottish diet: report of a working party to the Chief Medical Officer for Scotland. *Scotland's health: a challenge to us all?* Edinburgh: Scottish Office Home and Health Department, 1993
7. Medical Research Council Vitamin Study Group. Prevention of neural tube defects: results of the Medical Research Council vitamin study. *Lancet* 1991; **238**: 131–7
8. Department of Health. *Folic acid and the prevention of neural tube defects.* Report of an expert advisory group. London: Department of Health, 1992
9. White A, Freeth S, O'Brien M. *Infant feeding 1990.* Survey carried out by the Office of Population Censuses and Surveys for the Department of Health. London: HMSO, 1992
10. Howie PW, Forsyth JS, Ogston SA, Clark A, Florey CduV. Protective effect of breast feeding against infection. *British Medical Journal* 1990; **300**: 11–6
11. Calman KC. *On the state of the public health, 1993.* Annual report of the Chief Medical Officer of the Department of Health for the year 1993. London: HMSO, 1994
12. Department of Health. *Health of the nation: one year on—a report on the progress of the health of the nation.* London: Department of Health, 1993
13. Margetts B, Jackson AA. Interactions between people's diet and their smoking habits: the dietary and nutritional survey of British adults. *British Medical Journal* 1993; **307**: 1381–4

14. Nelson M, Bakaliou F, Trivedi A. Iron-deficiency anaemia and physical performance in adolescent girls from different ethnic backgrounds. *British Journal of Nutrition* 1994; **72**: 427–33

15. Hill AJ, Oliver S, Rogers PJ. Eating in the adult world: the rise of dieting in childhood and adolescence. *British Journal of Clinical Psychology* 1992; **31**: 95–105

16. Gregory J, Foster K, Tyler H, Wiseman M. *The dietary and nutritional survey of British adults.* London: HMSO, 1990

17. Adamson A, Rugg-Gunn A, Butler T, Appleton D, Hackett A. Nutritional intake, height and weight of 11–12 year old Northumbrian children in 1990 compared with information obtained in 1980. *British Journal of Nutrition* 1992; **68**: 543–63

18. Bailey AL, Finglas PM, Wright AJA, Southon S. Thiamin intake, erythrocyte transketolase activity and total erythrocyte thiamin in adolescents. *British Journal of Nutrition* 1994; **72**: 111–25

19. Anderson A, MacIntyre S, West P. Dietary patterns among adolescents in the West of Scotland. *British Journal of Nutrition* 1994; **71**: 111–22

20. Strain JJ, Robson PJ, Livingstone MBE, Primrose ED, *et al.* Estimates of food and macronutrient intake in a random sample of Northern Ireland adolescents. *British Journal of Nutrition* 1994; **72**: 343–52

21. Hackett AF, Rugg-Gunn AJ, Appleton DR, Eastoe JE, Jenkins GN. A 2-year longitudinal nutritional survey of 405 Northumberland children aged 11.5 years. *British Journal of Nutrition* 1984; **51**: 67–75

22. Armstrong N, Balding J, Gentle P, Kirby B. Patterns of physical activity among 11 to 16 year old British children. *British Medical Journal* 1990; **301**: 203–5

23. Department of Health, Committee on Medical Aspects of Food Policy. *Dietary reference values for food energy and nutrients for the United Kingdom.* Reports on Health and Social Subjects 41. London: HMSO, 1991

24. Godfrey KM, Redman CWG, Barker DJO, Osmond C. The effect of maternal anaemia and iron deficiency on the ratio of fetal weight to placental weight. *British Journal of Obstetrics and Gynaecology* 1991; **98**: 886–91

25. Valimiki MJ, Karkkainen M, Lamberg-Allardt C, Laitinen K, *et al.*, and the Cardiovascular Risk in Young Finns Study Group. Exercise, smoking, and calcium intake during adolescence and early adulthood as determinants of peak bone mass. *British Medical Journal* 1994; **309**: 230–5

26. National Task Force on Nutrition. *The balance of good health.* Health Education Authority, 1994

RCP REPORTS

Alcohol and the heart in perspective: sensible limits reaffirmed (1995)

Incontinence — Causes, management and provision of services (1995)

Provision of wheelchairs and special seating: guidance for purchasers and providers (1995)

Psychological care of medical patients — Recognition of need and service provision (1995)

Treatment of adult patients with renal failure: recommended standards and audit measures (1995)

Clinical audit scheme for geriatric day hospitals (1994)

Ensuring equity and quality of care for elderly people: the interface between geriatric and general internal medicine (1994)

Geriatric day hospitals: their role and guidelines for good practice (1994)

Good allergy practice (1994)

Homelessness and ill health (1994)

Part-time work in specialist medicine (1994)

Quality control in cancer chemotherapy: managerial and procedural aspects (1994)

Stroke audit package — produced by the UK Stroke Audit Group and the Royal College of Physicians (includes software) (1994)

Sleep apnoea and related conditions (1993)

Staff grade doctors: towards a better future (1993)

Reducing delays in cancer treatment — some targets (1993)

Allergy: conventional and alternative concepts (1992)

A charter for disabled people using hospitals (1992)

High quality long-term care for elderly people (1992)

Smoking and the young (1992)

Preventive medicine (1991)

A complete list of reports and other RCP publications is available from:

Publications Department, Royal College of Physicians
11 St Andrews Place, Regent's Park, London NW1 4LE

RCP PAPERBACKS

Health risks to the health care professional (1995)

Travel-associated disease (1995)

Psychiatric aspects of physical disease (1995)

Current themes in allergy and immunology (1994)

Regulation of the market in the National Health Service (1994)

Professional and managerial aspects of clinical audit (1994)

Management of stable angina (1994)

Access to health care for people from black & ethnic minorities (1993)

The role of hospital consultants in clinical directorates (1993)

Rationing of health care in medicine (1993)

Analysing how we reach clinical decisions (1993)

Current themes in rheumatology care (1993)

Measurement of patients' satisfaction with their care (1993)

Referrals to medical outpatients (1993)

Violence in society (1993)

Health systems and public health medicine in
the European Community (1992)

Measures of the quality of life (1992)

Current themes in diabetes care (1992)

Accidents and emergencies in childhood (1992)

Pharmaceutical medicine and the law (1991)

Paediatric specialty practice for the 1990s (1991)

Measuring the outcomes of medical care (1990)

A complete list of RCP publications is available from:

Publications Department, Royal College of Physicians
11 St Andrews Place, Regent's Park, London NW1 4LE